MALTHUS, MEDICINE, & MORALITY:

'MALTHUSIANISM' AFTER 1798

THE WELLCOME INSTITUTE SERIES IN THE HISTORY OF MEDICINE

Forthcoming Titles

Regenerating England:
Science, Medicine and Culture in Interwar Britain
Christopher Lawrence and Anna-K. Mayer

Women in Medicine
Lawrence Conrad and Anne Hardy (eds)

The Road to Medical Statistics
Eileen Magnello and Anne Hardy (eds)

'Captain of all these men of death'
The History of Tuberculosis in
Nineteenth and Twentieth Century Ireland
Greta Jones

Academic enquiries regarding the series should be addressed
to the editors C. J. Lawrence, V. Nutton and Roy Porter at
the Wellcome Institute for the History of Medicine,
183 Euston Road, London NW1 2BE, UK

MALTHUS, MEDICINE, & MORALITY:

'MALTHUSIANISM' AFTER 1798

edited by
Brian Dolan

Rodopi

Amsterdam – Atlanta, GA 2000

First published in 2000
by Editions Rodopi B. V., Amsterdam – Atlanta, GA 2000.

Brian Dolan © 2000

Design and Typesetting by Alex Mayor, the Wellcome Trust.
Printed and bound in The Netherlands by Editions Rodopi B. V.,
Amsterdam – Atlanta, GA 2000.

British Library Cataloguing in Publication Data
A catalogue record for this book is available from the British
Library
ISBN 90-420-0841-5 (Paper)
ISBN 90-420-0851-2 (Bound)

Malthus, Medicine & Morality:
'Malthusianism' After 1798 –
Amsterdam – Atlanta, GA:
Rodopi. – ill.
(Clio Medica 59 / ISSN 0045-7183;
The Wellcome Institute Series in the History of Medicine)

Front cover:
Lamech, holding a farm implement, points at a child; down in the street,
various acts of uninhibited licence go on. Engraving, sixteenth century.
Wellcome Library, London.

© Editions Rodopi B. V., Amsterdam – Atlanta, GA 2000

Printed in The Netherlands

All titles in the Clio Medica series (from 1999 onwards) are available to
download from the CatchWord website: http://www.catchword.co.uk

Contents

Acknowledgements

The inspiration for this volume came from a one-day symposium held in March 1998 at the Wellcome Institute for the History of Medicine, London. All of the contributors to this volume gave early versions of their papers at that meeting, with the exception of Timothy Alborn, who I was delighted to include here. My thanks to everyone. We thank the Wellcome Trust for the support to bring together this group in order to provide these critical perspectives on the history of Malthusianism and medicine. Finally, I would like to thank Alex Mayor at the Wellcome Trust for his expertise and efficiency in preparing this work for the press.

Notes on Contributors

Timothy L. Alborn is Assistant Professor of History at Lehman College, part of the City University of New York. He has published *Conceiving Companies: Joint-Stock Politics in Victorian England* (Routledge, 1998) and is working on a social history of British life assurance from 1840 to 1920.

Brian Dolan is Research Lecturer in the Wellcome Unit for the History of Medicine at the University of East Anglia. He is the author of *Exploring European Frontiers: British Travellers in the Age of Enlightenment* (Macmillan, 2000), and editor of *Science Unbound: Geography, Space & Discipline* (Umeå University Press, 1998). His next book, *Ladies of the Grand Tour*, will be published by HarperCollins in 2001.

Kathleen Gallagher-Kamper received her master's degree in Modern European History from the University of Notre Dame. She is currently working towards the completion of her Ph.D. on public policy and the Irish fever epidemic of 1817-1819. She is now teaching part-time in the History Department of LaSalle University, Philadelphia, PA.

Lesley Hall is Senior Assistant Archivist, Contemporary Medical Archives Centre, Wellcome Library for the History and Understanding of Medicine, and Honorary Lecturer in History of Medicine, University College London. Her publications include *Hidden Anxieties: Male Sexuality 1900-1950* (Oxford: Polity Press, 1991), and (with Roy Porter), *The Facts of Life: the creation of sexual knowledge in Britain, 1650-1950* (New Haven: Yale University Press, 1995). She is co-editor (with Franz Eder and Gert Hekma) of *Sexual Cultures in Europe 1: National Overviews* and *2: Themes in Sexuality* (Manchester: Manchester University Press, 1999). Forthcoming projects include an co-edited volume with Roger Davidson, *Sex, Sin, and Suffering: venereal diseases in the European social context since 1870* and a biography of Stella Browne (1880-1950), British socialist feminist sex radical.

Christopher Hamlin is Chair and Professor in the Department of History at the University of Notre Dame. He is author most recently of *Public Health and Social Justice in the Age of Chadwick, Britain 1800-1854* (Cambridge, 1998). His current research concerns the natural theology of public health in the nineteenth century.

Angus McLaren, professor of history at the University of Victoria, is the author of a number of books on the history of reproduction and sexuality. They include *Sexuality and Social Order: The Debate over the Fertility of Women and Workers in France, 1770-1920* (New York: Holmes and Meier, 1983), *Histoire de la contraception, tr. Isabella Morel et Jean Rosenthal* (Paris: Editions Noësis, 1996), and *Twentieth-Century Sexuality: A History* (Oxford: Blackwell, 1999).

Roy Porter is Professor of the Social History of Medicine at the Wellcome Institute for the History of Medicine in London. He is the author most recently of *The Greatest Benefit to Mankind: A Medical History of Humanity from Antiquity to the Present* (1997) and (with G.S. Rousseau) *Gout: The Patrician Malady* (1998).

Antonello La Vergata is professor of the History of Philosophy at the Universitàt della Calabria, Italy. His major publications include *Nonostante Malthus. Fecondit, popolazioni e armonia della natura, 1700-1900* (Turin: Bollati Boringhieri, 1990) and *Lìequilibrio e la guerra della natura. Dalla teologia naturale al darwinismo* (Naples: Morano, 1990), for which he was awarded in 1994 the Marc-Auguste Pictet Prize for the history of biology by the Société de Physique et de Histoire Naturelle de Geneve. He is the author of many articles in English, French, and Italian on the history of evolutionary theories, Darwinism, social Darwinism, theories of war and the relationship between biology and social theory.

Brian Young is a lecturer in Intellectual History at the University of Sussex. He is the author of *Religion and Enlightenment in Eighteenth-Century England* (Oxford: The Clarendon Press, 1998), and a co-editor of *History, Religion and Culture: British Intellectual History, 1750-1950* and *Economy, Polity and Society: British Intellectual History, 1750–1950* (Cambridge, C.U.P., 2000). He is currently at work on a study of empire, historiography and intellectual secularisation in the late eighteenth and early nineteenth centuries.

Robert M. Young is Professor of Psychotherapy and Psychoanalytic Studies at the Centre for Psychotherapeutic Studies, University of Sheffield. He is currently writing books on the concept of psychopatholoy and on sexuality. He has written a number of books and essays on Darwin, Darwinism, Malthusianism, and related matters in the history of biology and the human sciences, including *Mind, Brain, and Adaptation* (1970, 1990), *Darwin's Metaphor* (1985), *Mental Space* (1994), *Whatever Happened to Human Nature?* (in press). He is the editor of two quarterly journals, *Science as Culture* and *Free Associations*, co-editor of *Human Relations and Authority and Justice*, and associate editor of *Psychoanalytic Studies*.

Introduction: Malthusian Selections

Brian Dolan

Thomas Robert Malthus's reputation has lately been rehabilitated in the fields of social biology, demography, environmentalism, and economics, for diverse reasons and offering different results. Some recastings of the term 'Malthusianism' are intended to scare-monger: to resurrect the narrow thesis of 'misery and vice' that Malthus used when describing the consequences of 'unchecked' population growth. Others have used the term in a more prescriptive way, to recall Malthus's injunction of 'moral restraint', and urge that human survival depends on establishing morally-framed goals in which decisions about how to stabilise population, renew energy, conserve resources, and manage the future of genetic and environmental engineering are treated as matters of individual responsibility, but of global concern. Malthus is becoming second only to his most famous 'convert', Charles Darwin, as a nineteenth-century *agent provocateur* who is recast in the twentieth century as a malevolent harbinger of racist social and scientific theory.

In fact, the 'Darwin industry' has done much to raise Malthus's profile. A substantial literature has now been generated examining the extent to which Darwin's theory of natural selection was affected by Malthus's principle of organic superfecundity and the role classical political economists ascribed to 'competition'.[1] Robert M. Young has been one of the most outspoken scholars to explore the links between Darwin and Malthus.[2] In 'Malthus on Man – in Animals, No Moral Restraint', Young returns to reflect on the parallel extensions of 'Darwinian' biological and 'Malthusian' social discourses, and muses on the impact of their intellectual bequests on the fields of anthropology, moral philosophy, and on the modern rhetoric about biological fitness and environmentalism.

While there is not yet a 'Malthus industry' as such, increasing attention is turning to the reproduction and analysis of the Malthusian corpus. For example, scholars have gradually turned to closer readings of the six subsequent editions of his *Essay* to trace the further development of Malthus's argument and evidence. We now have readily available a number of different editions of Malthus's

1

Essay. Patricia James not only wrote the most thorough biography of Malthus to date, but prepared a detailed variorum edition of the *Essay*, published in 1989. Appendices to this useful edition – the core being a reprint of the second (1803) edition – reproduce re-written chapters and subtle variations in the content of different editions, contain explanatory editorial notes, and a comprehensive biographical register referring to Malthus's contemporaries and authorities.[3] Other recent reprints include the 'World's Classics' 1993 version of the first edition, edited by Geoffrey Gilbert, the Norton critical edition, and the facsimile reprints of the first and subsequent editions issued recently by Routledge/Thoemmes Press, to mention only a sample.[4] The increase in the number of reprints has also generated a number of scholarly studies that examine closely the narrative structure of Malthus's work. Scholars such as Donald Winch, Arthur Walzer, Salim Rashid, and perhaps most ambitiously, Samuel Hollander, being among the most critical modern readers.[5] This is not to mention the modern editions of other works by Malthus.[6]

Brian Dolan's 'Malthus's Political Economy of Health: the critique of Scandinavia in the *Essay on Population*' also looks at the changing design of Malthus's argument in later editions of the *Essay*, in this case focusing on the changes introduced in the second edition (1803). Malthus travelled on a 'fact-finding' mission to Scandinavia in 1799, where he sharpened his criticisms of over-reliance by the state on medical policy. This is clearly shown in Malthus's discussion of Sweden, where state-promotion of hospitals and free health care was attacked in the same vein as the English Poor Laws. By contrast, Norway's promotion of agriculture and education provided an example proving that 'misery and vice' need not necessarily prevail over population health.

Scandinavia was a valuable place to visit because of the dynamic political and social events in its countries in the latter half of the eighteenth century.[7] But the 'common context' of current events that influenced Malthus's – as well as his readers' – ideas about social welfare was much wider. The first edition of Malthus's fin-de-siècle tract – penned in an age of revolution and imperial anxiety – was an attack on the uncritical optimism of social and economic theorists who saw society moving towards inevitable future improvement and security. Malthus was early on highly sceptical of the increasing commercial and manufacturing interests of industrial society, just as he thought the government should be cautious in finding ways to root the economy in imperial projects or City investors should worry about the speculative propensities of businesses such as the East India

Company.[8] As Timothy Alborn's 'Boys to Men: Moral Restraint at Haileybury College' shows, Malthus's own concerns about imperial management were associated with his anxieties regarding the maintenance of morality as manifest by Britain's agents of empire. Thus Malthus, when professor at Haileybury College – the training ground for East India Company civil servants – applied his concept of 'moral restraint' to help discipline youthful students' unrestrained sexual desires and loose economic speculations.[9]

However theoretical or polemical Malthus's *Essay* was, it quickly found a wide readership. In an 1804 letter to an acquaintance in France, Thomas Jefferson wrote that he was giving his rarely found leisure moments over 'to the perusal of Malthus's work on population, a work of sound logic, in which some of the opinions of Adam Smith, as well as of the economists, are ably examined,' and went on to contrast Old and New World demographic conditions.[10] Even the British bluestocking Mary Berry found time while travelling around town in her chaise to read the *Essay* just months after its first publication, which she thought was 'uncommonly clearly thought and written, and contains much curious and uncontrovertible reasoning on the subject in question'.[11] The prose was seductive, but even in an emerging culture sympathetic to statistical laws, the fact-finding missionary of reproductive modification in fact was far from winning widespread acclaim for his accounts of nature's harsh handling of humanity. The immediate reactions by the professional classes, as three contributors to this volume show, were mixed.

Roy Porter's essay, 'The Malthusian Moment', places Malthus's physicalist and reductionist views on the human animal within the context of contemporary theories of medical materialism. Whatever Enlightenment sympathies there might have been towards Malthus's views of the natural biological economy, however, Porter's essay reveals that the earliest medics' responses to Malthus's 'principal conclusions' desired to place the blame on political mismanagement or Malthus's misguided reasoning rather than natural or providential necessity. To many medics, Malthus's ideas seemed to undermine their professional promise to improve public health. How could they, when their patients' progress was consigned to the dictates of Providence?[12] In 'Malthus and the Doctors: Political Economy, Medicine, and the State in England, Ireland, and Scotland, 1800-1840', Chris Hamlin and Kathleen Gallagher-Kamper show how the 'Malthusian' tendency of the human population to migrate towards inevitable ill-health was diversely interpreted, debated, or referred to other authorities by doctors. Using case studies from Ireland and

Scotland, Hamlin and Gallagher-Kamper show how Malthusian thinking was integrated into debates over poor laws, medical practices, and the moral probity of the population, though in ways that can be seen as either predominately medically or economically determined.

Perhaps the grand theories of population trends, natural laws, and Providential plans were simply matters of debate for those with different disciplinary directives. But it is hard to delineate boundaries of interest in Malthus's work: parliamentarians, political economists, and priests all dissected it for different reasons. Even Malthus's own vocational background was ranked according to how the reader felt most comfortable associating the author with the argument. As Brian Young points out in 'Malthus Among the Theologians', many of his critics responded to him as an Anglican clergyman as much as a political economist. It was no secret that elements of Malthus's theory, particularly his advocacy of 'moral restraint', were deemed unChristian and subject to theological censure. But, as Brian Young's essay shows, the theological responses to Malthus's work reveal an intriguing transition between the Cambridge liberalism of the later eighteenth century and the Evangelicalism of the early nineteenth.

As is clear from many of the essays in this volume, the persistence of the noun 'Malthusianism' over the last 200 years has a curious history. Its meanings have never been static. The term has certainly represented the pessimistic tenets of Malthus's political economy of natural resources, and of inevitable doom stemming from population growth of the sort stressed by contemporary reviewers when attacking his critique of the utopian philosophy of Condorcet and Godwin, or his apparent consignment of humanity to inevitable ill-health.[13] But few theories have provoked such divergent reactions. To Karl Marx, writing in 1867, the *Essay* was 'nothing more than a schoolboyish, superficial plagiary ... and does not contain a single sentence thought out by [Malthus] himself.' But to John Maynard Keynes, writing in 1933, it was 'a work of youthful genius' which could 'claim a place amongst those which have had great influence on the progress of thought.'[14] 'Malthusian checks' is a term now frequently used to mean what Malthus called 'positive checks' to population growth – instances of war, famine, and disease that he argued emerged and eliminated surplus populations that could not be sustained with the world's limited natural resources. The warnings of overpopulation issued by Malthus have been uncritically cited as historical and scientific underpinnings to twentieth-century debates on population, social medicine and welfare, birth control, support

4

for the developing world, and so on. He has been characterised as the 'sower of the seed of scientific racism,' and elsewhere the 'Malthusian' notion of surplus population has been treated as an economic concept masquerading as a biological problem.[15]

Strangely Malthus has been occasionally considered an early advocate of birth control. Elsewhere, and perhaps equally curiously, the figure of Malthus has loomed behind early twentieth-century pro-fornication arguments. So, the neo-Malthusian Percy Clark wrote in the *Birth Control Review* in 1925:

> If women are the ones primarily leading the present 'sex uproar', it is because they are fundamentally less prudish than men. ... Freedom of action on the part of women has brought with it a desire to attain the heights of love enjoyed by men, heights which could make Malthus, famous for his 'Essay on the Principle of Population', say, 'Perhaps there is scarcely a man who has once experienced the genuine delight of virtuous love ....'[16]

Reference to Malthus amongst neo-Malthusians served different, often celebratory or hagiographic, ends. To members of the 'Malthusian League', founded in 1877, for example, Malthus was a pioneer social activist as well as an eminent theorist. 'Malthus's fame is not the result of an accident', wrote John Maynard Keynes, President of the Malthusian League, at its fiftieth anniversary dinner in 1927. 'No one can read his famous book – particularly the first edition ... without appreciating that it is the fruit of a bold and eminent mind.' The programme for this dinner – which included Annie Besant, C.V. Drysdale (George's son), Margaret Sanger, and H.G Wells – included a chronology of the events that led to the foundation of the society over the previous hundred years (beginning with the 1832 publication of Knowlton's *The Fruits of Philosophy* that was banned and reprinted, leading to the Bradlaugh-Besant trial) and a colour chart of birth and death rates and infantile mortality in England and Wales. The speakers celebrated the achievements of Malthusianism. Alice Vickery, an honoured guest at the dinner, was referred to by Keynes as a woman for whom 'Malthusianism has always been an important part of the emancipation of women', and then he went on to give a biographical account of Malthus and an explanation of why they were 'sometimes called Neo-Malthusians.'[17]

Recent scholars have been much more sensitive and accurate in their analysis of Malthus's ideas regarding what he considered appropriate social and economic condition for reproduction, and factors individuals must weigh in choosing even to marry.[18] As Lesley

Hall shows in 'Malthusian Mutations: the Changing Politics and Moral Meanings of Birth Control in Britain', 'Malthusian' controls have been employed to refer euphemistically to the practice of artificial birth control. Hall examines Malthusianism as a recurrent element in the history of birth control in Britain rather than one particular phase which can be distinguished from others during which contraception was conceptualised as 'eugenics', 'birth control', 'family planning', and so on. In France, as Angus McLaren shows in 'Reproduction and Revolution: Paul Robin and Neo-Malthusianism in France', neo-Malthusian views were only propagated by Paul Robin and a small group of anarchists, but close analysis reveals that both neo-Malthusians and pro-natalists, usually seen as at odds, shared a number of concerns regarding differential fertility, degeneration, and the purported rise of perversions. Antonello La Vergata's essay in this volume, 'Biology and Sociology of Fertility: Reactions to the Malthusian Threat, 1798-1933', also looks at continental reactions to the 'Malthusian spectre.' La Vergata explores the 'providentialist-naturalist' version of anti-Malthusianism as extended into the socialist tradition (from utopian socialists to positivist socialists influenced by Herbert Spencer), drawing on examples from France, Germany, and Italy.

Malthus remains a controversial figure in history, and it seems likely that some will continue to hold him up as a champion of social and economic policy, while others will find new ways of taking him down with the various streams of philosophic thought that he appears inextricably linked to. The essays in this volume are certainly not intended to favour one portrait of Malthus over another, nor to re-define the 'essence' of 'Malthusianism.' Rather, it is hoped that they provide new historical perspectives on ways of re-contextualising, interlinking, and comparing themes central to Malthus, medicine, and morality over the last two hundred years.

Notes

1. See, for example, the discussion and bibliography in Scott Gordon, 'Darwin and Political Economy: The Connection Reconsidered', *Journal of the History of Biology* 22 (1989), 437-59.
2. See his reprinted essays in Robert M. Young, *Darwin's Metaphor: Nature's Place in Victorian Culture* (Cambridge: Cambridge University Press, 1985).
3. Thomas Robert Malthus, *An Essay on the Principle of Population; or, A view of its past and present Effects on Human Happiness; With an Enquiry into our Prospects respecting the future Removal or Mitigation*

of the Evils which it occasions, 2 vols, second edition (1803), Patricia
James (ed.) (Cambridge: Cambridge University Press, for the Royal
Economic Society, 1989), published with the variora of 1806, 1807,
1817, and 1826.

4. Malthus, *An Essay on the Principle of Population*, Geoffrey Gilbert
    (ed.) (Oxford: Oxford University Press, 1993); Philip Appleman
    (ed.) (New York: Norton, 1976); Samuel Hollander (ed.) (London:
    Routledge/Thoemmes Press, 1996).
5. Donald Winch, *Malthus* (Oxford: Oxford University Press, 1987);
    idem., 'Robert Malthus: Christian moral scientist, arch-demoralizer
    or implicit secular utilitarian?', *Utilitas* 5 (1993), 239-252; Arthur
    Walzer, 'Logic and Rhetoric in Malthus's *Essay on the Principle of
    Population*, 1798', *Quarterly Journal of Speech* 73 (1987), 1-17; Salim
    Rashid, 'Malthus's *Essay on Population*: The facts of "super-growth"
    and the rhetoric of scientific persuasion', *Journal for the History of
    Behavioural Sciences* 23 (1987), 22-36; Samuel Hollander,
    'Diminishing returns and Malthus's first *Essay on Population*: theory
    and application', *Écon Soc.* 23 (1989), 11-39; *idem.*, 'Malthus and
    Utilitarianism with Special References to the *Essay on Population*',
    Utilitas 1 (1989), 170-210; *idem.*, 'Malthus's Vision of the
    Population in the *Essay on Population*', *Journal for the History of
    Economic Thought* 12 (1990), 1-26; *idem.*, 'On Malthus's
    Physiocratic References', *History of Political Economy* 24 (1992), 369-
    80; also Geoffrey Gilbert, 'The Critique of Equalitarian Society in
    Malthus's *Essay*', *Phil. Soc. Sci.* 20 (1990), 35-55.
6. Malthus, *Principles of Political Economy: Variorum edition*, John
    Pullen (ed.), 2 vols (Cambridge: Cambridge University Press for the
    Royal Economic Society, 1989); E.A. Wrigley and David Souden
    (eds), *The Works of Thomas Robert Malthus*, 6 vols (London: William
    Pickering, 1986); for additional bibliographic guide, see also Samuel
    Hollander, 'New Editions of Malthus', *Utilitas* 3 (1991), 303-10;
    Salim Rashid, 'Recent literature on Malthus', in William Thweatt
    (ed.), *Classical Political Economy: A Survey of Recent Literature*
    (Boston: Kluwer Academic, 1988).
7. Brian Dolan, *Exploring European Frontiers: British Travellers in the
    Age of Enlightenment* (Basingstoke: Macmillan, 2000), chapter 2.
8. For a discussion of the uses of the 'four stages theory' of social
    development in economic thought, see R.L. Meek, *Social Science and
    the Ignoble Savage* (Cambridge: Cambridge University Press, 1976),
    particularly 222-25.
9. Philip Lawson, *The East India Company: A History* (London and
    New York: Longman, 1993), 129-130; C.A. Bayly, *Imperial*

Meridian: The British Empire and the World 1780-1830 (London and New York: Longman, 1989), 115.

10. Quoted in Dennis Hodgson, 'Images of Race and Responses to Malthus: The Study of Population in Antebellum America', unpublished paper presented at the American Sociological Association Annual Meeting, Washington, D.C., 1995.

11. Lady Theresa Lewis (ed.), *Extracts of the Journals and Correspondence of Miss Berry*, 3 vols (London: Longmans, Green, and Co., 1865), I, 73.

12. For dilemmas in the medical 'meanings' of sickness, see Roy Porter and Dorothy Porter, *In Sickness and in Health: The British Experience 1650-1850* (London: Fourth Estate, 1988), chapter 10.

13. For a collection of contemporary reviews, see Andrew Pyle (ed.), *Population: Contemporary Responses to Thomas Malthus* (Bristol: Thoemmes Press, 1994).

14. William Petersen, *Malthus* (London: Heinemann, 1979), 75; Robert Skidelsky, *John Maynard Keynes: A Biography: Volume 2: The Economist as Saviour, 1920-1937* (London: Macmillan, 1983).

15. Allen Chase, *The Legacy of Malthus: The Social Costs of the New Scientific Racism* (New York: Knopf, 1977); John Avery, *Progress, Poverty and Population: Re-reading Condorcet, Godwin and Malthus* (London: Cass, 1997).

16. Percy L. Clark, Jr., 'Is Love Worth Saving?', *Birth Control Review* 9 (1925), 42.

17. The programme and Keynes's remarks are from the Keynes Archive, King's College, Cambridge, PS/3/108 (programme), 118 ('notes on guests'), 111 ('Malthus in piam memoriam').

18. Alan Macfarlane, *Marriage and Love in England: Modes of Reproduction 1300-1840* (Oxford: Basil Blackwell, 1986), chapters 1-3; Simon Szreter, *Fertility, Class, and Gender in Britain 1860-1940* (Cambridge: Cambridge University Press, 1996).

1

Malthus's Political Economy of Health:
The Critique of Scandinavia in the *Essay on Population*

Brian Dolan

1998 was the 200th anniversary of the publication of the first edition
of Malthus's *Essay on the Principle of Population*. 1999 was the 250th
anniversary of the foundation of what became the National Central
Bureau of Statistics in Sweden. The year after the publication of the
first edition of the *Essay*, Malthus, *the* historical demographer of his
epoch, travelled to Sweden: *the* land where the question of
population was paramount. This trip, part of his broader
Scandinavian tour, enabled Malthus to draw on the world's oldest
systematically recorded statistics on birth, marriage, and mortality
rates which added significantly to the empirical data that
underpinned his theory of population espoused in the second and
subsequent editions of his *Essay*.

Malthus's Scandinavian trip was not a leisurely Grand Tour but a
fact-finding mission organised by Edward Daniel Clarke, Malthus's
colleague from Jesus College, Cambridge, who had already spent
most of the 1790s travelling around Britain and southern Europe
with patrician students. The plans for the Scandinavian tour were
particularly fitting for Clarke and Malthus since both wished to
gather information about current affairs in the northern states.
Looking at Malthus's travels and the way his empirical data affected
his later political philosophy provides a way to contrast different
opinions of various travellers regarding government patronage of
science and medicine and also the different ways that the experience
of travel was used to support their theoretical assumptions of what
defined 'modern' European states.

Malthus's interests in Scandinavia concerned, in broadest terms,
the 'health' of the economy, agrarian production, and population
reproduction. The health of the economy affected the health of the
population, and the political management of the land affected both,
because of population's reliance on agriculture. As befitted the
philosophies of national improvement and political progress,

economic questions became integral to broader concerns about the condition of civil society. Scandinavia was a profitable place to visit for comparative analysis in statistics and demography, medicine, public health programmes, agrarian improvement, and evangelical philanthropy.

In Sweden, scholarship in social and economic life continued to develop in the eighteenth century as the study of 'cameralistics'; this included state finance, administrative law, estate management, and agricultural economics. In the mid-eighteenth century, the science of cameralistics was being coupled with population studies to collect practical data in order to evaluate prospects for future economic improvement. The professor of economics at Uppsala University, Anders Berch, especially promoted the collection of practical statistics. In his *On Studying the Wealth of Nations by Political Arithmetic* (1746), Berch wanted to conduct a quantitative analysis of contemporary society and evaluate the nation's capital strength relative to its population, natural resources, manufactures, consumption, and so on, in order to determine how they affected social equilibrium. Berch became one of the first to calculate the size of Sweden's population. Shortly after, however, Pehr Elvius, the Secretary of the Royal Swedish Academy of Sciences (which had for some time supported the need to acquire vital statistics) used data on birth and mortality rates, and life expectancy, to independently conclude that the population was much lower.[1]

It is generally recognised that demographic data was becoming widely collected in the eighteenth century and used to compute prices of annuities, life insurance, and population statistics.[2] But in 1749, Sweden in particular embraced the 'quantifying spirit' by instituting an official policy requiring local pastors to collect, at five-year intervals, data on birth and mortality rates, along with marriage statistics (known as the *Tabellverket*). In 1756 this became the Statistical Committee (called the *Tabellkommissionen*), which was the forerunner to the Central Bureau of Statistics (1858).[3] This gives Sweden (which included Finland until 1809) the oldest demographic records in the world. By the time of Malthus's visit, the records were gaining international renown, and had already been commented upon by other travellers. William Coxe, for example, summarised trends in Sweden's population growth and discussed the work of the '*Tabell Commission*', and reproduced tables of birth and mortality rates. Clarke also separately noted that statistics was the most cultivated science, and mused at the profits that Malthus would reap during his tour.[4] As will be further discussed below, the government used these records to promote arguments about the need to increase population. An optimistic plan, promoted by mercantilist economists, proposed that through population growth and public health measures, the wealth and power of the state would grow. As we will see, Malthus had different views. But before entering into further discussion of his critique, it is worthwhile illuminating the relevant context of debates about social improvement.

Condorcet, Godwin, and the perfectibility of humankind

Mercantilist optimism affected another philosophy of human progress and perfectibility espoused by the so-called 'utopians'. The eighteenth-century utopian philosophers believed that in a perfectly organised society, a population of any size would be able to share its available resources and avoid imposing government controls or policing of property for the equal distribution of subsistence. After the outbreak of the French Revolution, questions of the perfectibility of human kind, equality, government control over natural resources, and so on, gained political potency, and an array of 'scientific' judgements about the history and progress of civilisation were used to analyse contemporary social conditions. In this context, the Marquis de Condorcet in France espoused a utopian philosophy. During the Reign of Terror in 1794, Condorcet, under proscription from Robespierre and in hiding, wrote the work for which he is best know, the *Esquisse d'un tableau historique des progrès de l'esprit humain* (1795; *Sketch for an Historical Picture of the Progress of the Human Mind*). In it, he proposed that the human race had gone through great 'epochs' of history, in which humans have been in continuous progress from a state of savagery through levels of increasing enlightenment and happiness. In a future epoch, he argued, inequality between nations, classes, and ultimately individuals would be eliminated, and humans would enjoy intellectual, moral, and physical perfection.[5]

The English social philosopher and political journalist William Godwin had expressed a similarly optimistic view of the future perfectibility of humankind. In his *An Enquiry Concerning Political Justice, and Its Influence on General Virtue and Happiness* (1793), Godwin advanced a doctrine of extreme individualism, arguing that small self-subsisting groups should replace large government and social institutions to ensure the future improvement of society. In his radical philosophy, he argued that all forms of social organisation (judicial, religious, educational, etc.) were oppressive, and after their removal humankind would be liberated from misery, ignorance, and poverty, and live in a world of uncoerced morality, virtue, and happiness. Godwin anticipated a potential population problem, and predicted that humans would 'probably cease to propagate' and 'perhaps be immortal' after their liberated rationality eliminated sexual passions.

Malthus's view was quite different. Where Condorcet and Godwin entertained visions of progress, peace, and plenitude, Malthus focused on population problems, poverty, and public policy. He believed that population growth would inevitably exceed levels of subsistence necessary for survival. His views were largely compatible with the philosophy of the 'physiocrats', who believed that a nation's wealth was attributable to agricultural productivity, and that population growth itself would not lead to increased wealth. The physiocrats objected to pronatalism, arguing that human reproduction could not be encouraged to a point beyond that sustainable without widespread poverty. They also objected to any other strategies involving the intervention of the government to promote population growth, leading to the pronouncement of their famous *laissez-faire* policy that became so influential to the thinking of later classical economists. After reading Condorcet and Godwin in 1797, Malthus concluded that the notion of a perfectible society was a theory built on sand.

Malthus wrote the first edition of his *Essay* as a critique of the utopian theories of Condorcet and Godwin, and criticised what he considered their unsound principles of reasoning. He attacked Condorcet's theory of the 'indefinite' perfectibility of humankind for being entirely speculative, ambiguous, and devoid of proper methods of investigation and authenticated proofs. The future epoch envisioned by Condorcet might have been a noble dream, but it was unrealistic to suppose that the capacity for biological improvement had no limits.[6]

Similarly, Godwin's fanciful notions of human 'immortality', the proscription of all emotions and passions, and the pervasive control of the mechanisms of rationality were inventions of the imagination. True, reason was the proper corrective to the impulse to overindulge in sensual pleasures, but the mind could never triumph over the physical condition. The pressures of an ever-increasing population checked the route to Condorcet's 'perfectibility of man' as well as Godwin's 'immortal man'; the attainment of a sovereign intellect was checked by bodily cravings. How, then, to balance growing numbers with available resources to remedy perpetual cravings? Godwin's thought regarding the increase in human population, which he conceded could take place for 'myriads of centuries' before perfectibility, was merely that 'There is a principle in human society, by which population is perpetually kept down to the level of the means of subsistence.' But what was that principle? Malthus's *Essay* of 1798 was his forthright attempt to answer this question.[7]

The Essays on population

It is an oft-cited asseveration that Malthus's *Essay* was a pessimistic, harsh, gloomy treatise where humanity's future was consigned to the discouraging forces of nature. And, indeed, even Malthus recognised that his attack on utopian thinking and the amount of space he took to dwell on the existence of 'misery and vice' made him appear overtly despairing of the human condition. His main argument concerned two main premises: first, population, when unchecked, grows at a geometrical ratio, doubling itself every twenty-five years or so. Subsistence, on the other hand, which meant the minimum standard of living and the amount of food necessary to the life of a human, increases only in an arithmetical ratio – in uniform incremental increases. Thus, population would quickly exceed levels of subsistence, which meant that the surplus population would face war, starvation, and death. Such catastrophic consequences to a rapidly growing population were rather misleadingly referred to as 'positive' checks. But Malthus argued that such dire ends could be avoided if humans exercised 'preventative' checks to population growth: prevention of marriage and procreation.

Much of the contemporary criticism that Malthus received stemmed from a pervading sense of vulnerability in a Europe rocked with political turmoil. It was an age of revolution and local unrest. Malthus wrote in the wake of the American and French Revolutions; Napoleon's armies were running rampant on the Continent; and unruly mobs in London were protesting the high price of food, forcing William Pitt to propose an amendment to the Poor Laws which would provide additional support for labourers. These were not conditions favourable to the reception of a treatise that warned of war, disease, and pestilence. Yet, Malthus hoped people would heed the warnings, and take necessary action in order to prevent collision with nature's destructive forces.

The first essay was written as a polemic. It contained the premises of his theory about the balance of population and subsistence, but presented little supporting evidence. To argue the existence of population checks, he discussed the fluctuations in populations of ancient society, and amongst primitive peoples, tribal communities, and nations of shepherds, Indians, Hottentots and hunters. Cursory remarks about the states in modern Europe declared that population was growing, but more slowly due to the implementation of preventative checks – the result of rational foresight of the difficulties involved with rearing a family amongst the labouring classes.[8]

But Malthus was also concerned about the happiness and health of the human population, and shared the Enlightenment view that social improvement and progress needed rational management. His was a philosophy of scarcity and finitude: progress had limits, economic and ecological resources were finite; benevolence (philanthropy, medical aid, and charity) must be regulated. As natural theologians such as Johann Süssmilch (whom Malthus cited) or William Paley (whom Malthus considered one of his most influential converts) had shown, apparent regularities in birth and mortality rates could be used to show that oscillations in population were part of God's design. Wars and famine were not written into the fabric of population health, but morality and rationality should be used to prevent these 'positive' checks. If resources could not be increased, then population reproduction must be diminished. There was not enough food to go around at nature's feast; scarcity was ordained by providence to stimulate hard work, health, and happiness. 'Parson Malthus' espoused moral improvement and civic responsibility, and argued that problems were challenges to be overcome: 'Evil exists in the world, not to create despair, but activity.'[9]

Despite Malthus's last-minute assurances of hope rather than despair, his critics remained sceptical. Some reviewers, Malthus thought, considered the essay 'a specious argument inapplicable to the present state of society' since it departed from preconceived opinion.[10] Malthus was intent, when preparing the second edition of it, to demonstrate its applicability to modern society. Two years after writing the first edition, he wrote:

> I have deferred giving another edition of it in the hope of being able to make it more worthy of public attention, by applying the principle directly and exclusively to the existing state of society, and endeavouring to illustrate the power and universality of its operation from the best authenticated accounts that we have of the state of other countries.[11]

He wanted his 'principle of population' to be accepted as natural law, with all the universality in its application and constancy which characterises scientific fact. This required empirical evidence and demonstrable proof. He needed first-hand experience of the condition of modern states, and a journey to Scandinavia provided the perfect opportunity to gather population facts. Concerns over population maintenance, government assistance to the poor, notions of progress in society, health of civic and political bodies, all bear on his philosophy and his observations when travelling to Scandinavia.

Population Health: Norway and Sweden

Before travelling, Malthus had some preconceived ideas about what he might find in Scandinavia. In the first edition of his *Essay*, it had entered discussion in reference to population statistics on 'Sweden, Norway, Russia, and the kingdom of Naples' briefly cited in Richard Price's opus on birth and mortality rates, which was used to recommend premiums for life insurance and annuities. Multiple editions of Price's work were published at the end of the eighteenth century, but knowledge of the 'Swedish tables' remained little until Malthus's visit.[12] However, the *availability* of statistical resources was inviting to Malthus, who saw in them an opportunity to hammer out laws of population growth the way Süssmilch had done in his natural theological account of the *Development of the Human Race*, which Malthus also learned about from Price (who cited Süssmilch's tables).[13] The structure of the second edition of the *Essay* reveals the extent to which his journey to Scandinavia and the compilation of data from other sources assisted his argument.

The new *Essay* was divided into four 'books', all published as part of one quarto volume. The first book examined the checks to population in antiquity and amongst savage peoples, including the Greeks and Romans, pastoral nations, and the American Indians. Relying on a bevy of travellers' narratives, he reiterated the existence of polygamy in Africa, incessant war in the 'Kossacks', and promiscuity amongst the South Sea islanders. The checks in the 'barbarous' nations were positive, resulting in cannibalism, famine, plague, epidemic and endemic maladies. Misery was caused by vice, which sealed the condemned fate of the barbarians. But people in modern Europe had a chance. The 'civilised man hopes to enjoy, the savage expects only to suffer'.[14] Hopes of happiness would only materialise if proper preventative measures were taken to balance population growth and its subsistence.

Malthus's liberal use of travel literature which discussed distant parts of the world enabled him to pack detail into his principle. Travel books were resources frequently tapped by social theorists looking for empirical data about different cultures. The round-the-world *Voyages* of Bougainville and Captain Cook were already widely used by writers such as Locke, Rousseau, Montesquieu, and others looking for descriptions that characterised the non-European.[15] But Malthus intended to be most persuasive by using his own travel narratives to analyse the condition of *modern Europe*. A discussion of the Scandinavian and northern countries thus formed the entirety of book two of the second edition, a critical place within the significantly revised structure. 'In reviewing the states of modern Europe', began book two, 'we shall be assisted in our inquiries by registers of births, deaths, and marriages, which, when they are complete and correct, point out to us with some degree of precision whether the prevailing checks to population are of the positive or preventative kind'.[16] His travel diaries reveal the extent of his Scandinavian tour – trekking north through Norway to Trondheim, and returning along the Norwegian-Swedish borders – as well as information on the customs, produce, and, of course, population that was gleaned through interviews with anyone from peasant to prince.[17] Malthus polished his prose, and moved much of the material directly into his new chapters on Scandinavia, giving the *Essay* the flavour of a first-hand, empirically proved, account of the applicability of the principle. This was the 'best authenticated account' he could offer.

Malthus stated that the powerful tendency for population to increase applied as much to northern Europe as anywhere, but that particular kinds of preventative checks have prevailed to keep population under control. What were these preventative checks? Norway and Sweden provided two different models, useful for comparison.

In Norway, certain factors affected mortality rates. Malthus observed that in the eighteenth century, Norway was 'peculiarly exempt from the drains of people by war', and that the Nordic climate was 'remarkably free from epidemic sickness'. As a result, the 'mortality is less than in any other country in Europe', 1 to 48, as shown in the Norwegian census which had begin in 1769. This was also close to the figure given by the former Professor of Statistics in Copenhagen, Frederik Thaarup, who Malthus met in Norway and discussed 'the causes that had impeded or promoted the population of Norway'.[18] Malthus's assessment of the unusually favourable effects of the climate appear to be supported by a number of contemporary Scandinavian writers, as summarised recently by Karin Johannisson:

The cold protected the people from infectious diseases and made them 'merry, lively, and manly'. The snow on the ground prevented nutritious substances from evaporating and, when it melted transformed the rotting leaves and needles into rich humus. The woods were teeming with useful game – 'if anyone seriously tried to domesticate our moose, they might well become our camels' –and lakes and rivers were swarming with salmon and other splendid fish, pearl-filled molluscs, oysters, and lobsters. ... They were spared from the burning sun of hotter countries 'where the people, drained by the heat, for much of the year must splash around all day in their water barrels'. They could walk in the forests without fear of tigers, lions, leopards and apes and they could fish in lakes and rivers without being frightened by dreadful hippopotamuses and bloodthirsty crocodiles. Given persevering application, all this splendour would show a wonderful capacity to multiply. 'When wilderness and wastes are cultivated, a whole new land will be created, much more fruitful than this, milder in climate, more pleasant in every way, rich and able to support and feed many million people more than now.'[19]

Malthus's reading of the Scots physician Thomas Short further confirmed some of the different ways that cold and warm climates affect health. Citing Short's 1000 page tome, *A General Chronological History of the Air, Water, Seasons ...*, he discussed how warm, southern, populous countries cannot often endure drought, suggesting that insufficient food supplies can go bad, 'producing epidemics, either in the shape of great ravaging plagues, or of less violent, but more constant, sickness'. In cold countries, on the contrary, the 'antiseptic quality of the air' alleviated misery that could arise from insufficient or bad food.[20]

While the climate appeared to possess qualities that might help prevent the propagation of disease, it was also an obstacle that a healthy population must overcome. The northern environment, while 'antiseptic', was also harsh. Malthus noted that because such little soil area was capable of being cultivated for fruitful agricultural return, and because the northern seasons were so short, sudden and unexpected changes in the climate inevitably had devastating effects on the well being of the labouring classes. In seasons of drought and bad harvests, such as the occasion when Malthus travelled to Scandinavia in summer 1799, the majority of the population resorted to adding the inner bark of pine to their bread for sustenance for the following winter. Even in better times, conditions were harsh. The arable land was hard to till, the soil was rocky, and the mountains made cattle farming difficult. But the Norwegians did not lack spirit for agricultural labour. Their physique displayed evidence of their arduous work. He noted that the 'Norwegians in general have appeared to us as if they were well fed. The women have plump round faces; & most of the boys who have been with us to take back the horses have been very good looking lads, & stouter & with better calves to their legs than those of the same age in England.'[21]

For Malthus, a commitment to agricultural labour reinforced a spirit of survival, and lead to moral improvement and healthiness. Eric Pontoppidan described the self-sufficient Norwegian farmers as 'polypragmatic peasants', whose work, which involved tanning, weaving, carpentry, joining, shoemaking, and other regular duties, was a largely undifferentiated labour force which retained a spirit of communal responsibility and mutual aid.[22] In his travel diary, Malthus noted the opinion of a Norwegian gentleman that attention to the improvement in agriculture was a primary concern in Norway. 'One of the most powerful reasons of the present prosperity of the country he thought was, that the people now depended less on fishing, & more upon the produce of the earth.'[23]

Agricultural resourcefulness was the driving force to a better society. Necessity commanded efficiency; producing food helped keep at bay nature's afflicting visitations. Of course, the rich could live in the Malthusian world of scarcity, indulge in profligate spending, and invest in manufactures.[24] But social progress for the masses was different. For the working classes who formed the subjects of Malthus's essay, husbandry was the lifeblood of the economy. Thus Malthus's criticism of Hume of the apparent advantages of the transfer of economic resources from agriculture to the new class of manufacturers:

> Agriculture is not only, as Hume states, that species of industry which is chiefly requisite to the subsistence of multitudes, but is in fact the sole species by which multitudes can exist; and all the numerous arts and manufactures of the modern world, by which such numbers appear to be supported, have no tendency whatever to increase the population, except so far as they tend to increase the quantity and to facilitate the distribution of the products of agriculture.[25]

For Malthus, the new manufacturing trades were an appendage to the economy that supplanted productive labour, and gave in to a growing commodity culture which was fed by what Adam Smith called 'mankind's insatiable appetite for trinkets and baubles'.[26] His argument here was reminiscent of the physiocrats' distinction between three social orders: the productive agricultural labourers, the proprietors of land, and the unproductive ('sterile') manufacturers. Only the agricultural labourers yielded real value to society.[27] In a country, such as Norway, that concentrated labour in agriculture, the lower classes were provided with a more comfortable lot in life than might be expected in the harsh northern climate. 'There is nothing in the climate, or the soil, that would lead to the supposition of its being in an extraordinary manner favourable to the general health of the inhabitants', wrote Malthus. Nevertheless, Norway had one of the lowest mortality rates in Europe. 'It may be said, perhaps, with some truth, that one of the principle reasons of the small mortality in Norway is that the tows are inconsiderable and few, and that few people are employed in unwholesome manufactures.'[28] Urban manufacturers created idle wealth, and ran the risks of going out of fashion, suddenly removing the security of lifestyle that could accommodate early marriages and family planning. Critical as Malthus sounds, he should not be interpreted as rejecting manufacturing economy outright. Writing in the age of industrialisation, he recognised that through the commercialisation and mechanisation of agriculture, the vast advances made in agricultural production in the eighteenth century could be further developed. By creating an economy where farms became rural factories, population fears might be alleviated.[29]

So far, Malthus's observations of Norway suggest that lack of *positive* checks and a climate that induced hard work provided for a reasonably healthy population.[30] But there also existed further *preventative* checks, which were crucial to maintaining a healthy population. These checks concern the rigorous social control exercised by local parishes over marriages, and particular working conditions that affected labourers earning enough to support a family.

He found that the marital age was late in Norway, and he attributed this to military and civil institutions. In his travel diaries, Malthus recorded a conversation where he had been informed that:

> Every man in Denmark & Norway born of a farmer or labourer is a soldier. Those born of sailors are sailors. Formerly the officer of the district might take them at any age he pleased and he generally preferred a man from 25 to 30 to those that were younger. After being taken the man could not marry without producing a certificate signed by the minister of the parish that he had substance

enough to support a wife & family, & even then it was at the will of the officer to let him marry or not. This, & the uncertainty in respect to the time of being taken has hitherto operated as a strong preventative check to population in Norway, & accounts for their increasing so slowly, tho people live so long.[31]

The laws of consignment and the discretionary powers of the military officers had changed by the time Malthus visited Norway, and more liberties were given to soldiers to marry. However, 'many are of opinion that that the peasants will now marry too young, and that more children will be born than the country can support'.[32] To guard against this, the local parish continued to impose regulations over marriage, giving the priest the power to refuse marrying a couple thought not to be adequately prepared. Custom prevailed to discourage early marriage.

Due to the self-sufficiency of the rural economy and the nature of the division of property, additional caution was exercised for want of economic security. Each village had its own number of peasants that provided the labour more than equal to the demand, and employment was strictly regulated, compelling labourers to wait until an opportunity arose to rear a family. Larger farms could employ 'house-men', a married labourer who, in return for lower wages, was given a plot of property sufficient to maintain a family.

> Except in the immediate neighbourhood of the towns, and on the seacoast, a vacancy of a place of this kind is the only prospect which presents itself of providing for a family. From the small number of people, and the little variety of employment, the subject is brought distinctly within the view of each individual; and he must feel the absolute necessity of repressing his inclinations to marriage till some such vacancy offer.[33]

The surveillance of the local parish, the traditional custom of caution over premature marriage, and the limited opportunities of employment were preventative checks to population growth. Awareness of personal responsibilities, 'repressing inclinations to marriage', amounted to what Malthus termed 'moral restraint'. The phrase referred to restraint from marriage for prudential reasons, and not followed by 'irregular gratifications ... promiscuous intercourse, unnatural passions, violations to the marriage bed, and improper acts to conceal the consequence of irregular connexions'.[34] While this term to describe this preventative check was introduced in the second edition of the *Essay*, suggestions of moral restraint appear in the first.[35]

To marry without prospects was immoral. The concept was used to argue that moral responsibility, which was linked to marriage restraint and hard work, was an avenue which led to population control without nature's harsh 'positive' checks. His chapter on Norway was offered as a warning about the effects of early marriages on population explosions, and proof of the efficacy of moral restraint.[36]

Malthus was full of praise for Norway's management of population and natural resources. 'Norway is, I believe, almost the only country in Europe where a traveller will hear any apprehensions expressed of a redundant population, and where the danger to the happiness of the lower classes of people from this cause is, in some degree, seen and understood.'[37] It was a country perfectly prepared to accept the dangers of the principle of population, and undertook acceptable measures to ensure they maintained a healthy and happy society.

If Norway was the place for the Malthusian 'utopia', then Sweden represented the Malthusian 'dystopia'. One striking contrast was that employment in agriculture was not so complete in Sweden as it was in Norway. That, he concluded, explained why 'the positive check has operated with more force, or the mortality has been greater' in Sweden.[38] Despite their similar climate, Norway's population was more healthy than in Sweden: in the former, the people wore 'faces of plenty and content', in the latter they were 'absolutely starving'.[39] This boiled down to fundamental differences in government attitudes and administration over the maintenance of the health of the population. The prevailing defect was the 'continual cry of the government for an increase of subjects, [which tended] to press the population too hard, against the limits of subsistence, and consequently to produce diseases which are the necessary effect of poverty and bad nourishment'.[40]

As mentioned briefly above, the Swedish government was keen to collate population statistics in order to determine the rate of population growth and health. The concern over collecting demographic statistics was rooted in a dominating mercantilist economic philosophy. This emphasised that accelerating population growth would lead to an increase in the nation's economic wealth and political power. More people created more demand, and more productive labour to exploit natural resources, pay taxes, and defend the nation. Encouraging immigration and preventing emigration, and stimulating nativity amongst the working classes would increase population. Pronatalist policies assisted by advocating marriage and procreation, stressing liberal reforms of sexual morality, and imposing tax penalties and social stigma on those who failed to enlarge their families.[41] Justification for mercantilist population theory could, and often did, refer to the biblical injunction to 'be fruitful and multiply'. Most were not concerned with possible adverse effects of population growth, being confident that any level of population would be capable of securing appropriate levels of subsistence.

Malthus disagreed. Like Norway, Sweden was not by default an unhealthy country, but, he argued, it was prone to unfavourable ('positive') checks to population for reasons relating to agricultural investment and their promotion of public health. First, Sweden was overly dependent upon their own agricultural production, neglecting assistance that could be gained through importation or more concentrated efforts for agricultural improvement. This resulted in particularly 'unhealthy years', when the harvest season was adversely affected by the climate. Here Malthus benefited from the demographic statistics, the 'bookkeeping of life and death', that had been collected since 1749.[42]

When Malthus visited Stockholm after leaving Norway, he met the Uppsala University mathematician Henrik Nicander, who was Secretary to the Royal Swedish Academy of Sciences. Nicander, who corresponded with the Swiss statistician Leonhard Euler and Condorcet, was also Secretary to the *Tabellkommission*. His *magnum opus* on Swedish population statistics from 1772 to 1795 was just beginning to be published when Malthus visited him, and was not completely in print until 1802. With Nicander, Malthus had the opportunity to see first-hand the elephant portfolios which contain the collated data sent from local parishes, and to discuss the work of Nicander's predecessor as Secretary to the Academy, Per Wilhelm Wargentin, and his correspondents, Süssmilch and Richard Price.[43]

After his visit to Stockholm and through continued correspondence with Nicander and others such as Thaarup, Malthus was able to use these unique statistics to demonstrate the correlation between mortality decreases and increases during respective years of good and bad harvests. Of course, in searching for supporting data, the theory itself somewhat predetermined which statistics would be chosen for illustrations. A number of different theories can find 'factual' support if they draw from a large enough statistical bank. As has been pointed out, Malthus was fairly sloppy with some details, ignoring context and distorting figures at times. This can partly be accounted for by poor translations, printing errors, and misinformation passed verbally, but Malthus himself was not bothered, and preferred 'illustrative examples' to facts.[44] He interpreted the data in light of his theory, and asked others to interpret his theory in light of the figures. In the case of Sweden, the data 'clearly proved' that in Sweden, as elsewhere, population has a tendency to increase, but that, because Sweden lacked an efficient system of agriculture, there quickly emerged a poorly nourished, redundant and unhealthy population. Thus, the increase in population was solely 'productive of misery'.[45] A fruitful remedy could be the improvement of the political regulations of agricultural production, most profitably leading to better knowledge of crop rotation, and of fertilising their lands. Instead, it appeared to Malthus that the Swedish government was pursuing the misguided course of attempting to treat the sick rather than address the cause of sickness.

In Sweden, medical concerns were intimately bound to population questions, and therefore to political and economic issues. The health of the country was reflected in the health of its population, and the government hoped that medical aid would help encourage the growing numbers of people. To hope that medical care would act as a steroid for population statistics was sanguine indeed. Medical care in the eighteenth century was of limited assistance in dealing with most ailments, as medical knowledge was often deficient and skilled practitioners were few and far between. But the establishment of the 'cause of death' category as part of the population statistics and its applications in the *Collegium Medicum* (an incipient National Board of Health) through the activities of doctors such as Abraham Bäck, helped remedy the situation.[46]

By the end of the eighteenth century, Sweden had established a strong, state-supported framework for public health, which rapidly advanced to include expanding medical education, prevention campaigns, and free medical services. Medical assistance was centrally regulated and care distributed amongst different categories of sick, poor, and disabled. Portions of enlightenment philosophy espoused that surveillance and rational cooperative action could prove effective for improving public health. Such reasoning informed the theoretical system of 'medical police' that was elaborated by the Habsburg physician Johann Peter Frank, which was reflected in the paternalistic political philosophy of cameralism.[47] Frank's ideas were disseminated at Uppsala University by the professor of political economy, Anders Berch. While Frank's ideas were not put into practice, health care in Sweden was closely bound to state action, with the government keen to protect health for its own selfish ends.[48]

When the demographic data began to pile up, the Swedish

Parliament reflected on the figures and solicited the opinion of the *Collegium Medicum* about the mortality rates. In a number of reports to Parliament, the *Collegium Medicum* argued that a high percentage of deaths could be avoided if the state, in whose interests the preservation of labouring and tax-paying lives would largely benefit, created conditions favourable to the propagation of medical officers and institutional health services.[49] In 1752, when the *Collegium Medicum* was first approached by Parliament about the demographic records, the first hospital was opened in Stockholm, and throughout the rest of the eighteenth century over twenty others sprouted around the country.

Malthus was critical of these developments. He believed that establishing lying-in and foundling hospitals for the care of infants was wasted money. While he acknowledged that in some particular circumstances the establishment of colleges of medicine could prove 'extremely beneficial', he quickly recited his outspoken opinion on the subject:

> Lying-in hospitals, as far as they have an effect, are probably rather prejudicial than otherwise as, according to the principle on which they are generally conducted, their tendency is certainly to encourage vice. Foundling hospitals, whether they attain their professed and immediate object or not, are in every view hurtful to the state.[50]

Elsewhere he was equally austere in his judgement. One of the main reasons for premature mortality, he argued, was that these institutions, 'miscalled philanthropic', diffused individual responsibility toward families and health. High mortality rates which exist in countries with rely on hospital care 'appears to me incontrovertibly to prove that the nature of these institutions is not calculated to answer the immediate end that they have in view, which I conceive to be the preservation of a certain number of citizens to the state, who might otherwise, perhaps, perish from poverty or false shame.'[51] Foundling hospitals appeared to present proofs that parents were unable to support their families, and, worse still, the hospitals themselves were largely unsuccessful in keeping children alive. His dire conclusion was that establishing hospitals of this kind appeared to be the most effective way to create positive checks to population.

Foundling hospitals were disagreeable because it relieved parents of responsibility that was vital to proper human development. The remitted attention of institutions in place of the mother's fostering care was detrimental to the infant. In addition, it was unjust to other members of society since, as with other state-supported medical aid or poor relief, it relieved some in society of civil responsibility and concentrated care in a few at the expense of the rest. Malthus's bitter critique of Swedish health care was argued in the same vein as his attack on the English poor laws where he was unequivocal:

> The poor-laws of England tend to depress the general condition of the poor in these two ways. Their first obvious tendency is to increase population without increasing the food for its support. A poor man may marry with little or no prospect of being able to support a family in independence. They may be said therefore in some measure to create the poor which they maintain. ... Secondly, the quantity of provisions consumed in workhouses upon a part of the society, that cannot in general be considered as the most valuable part, diminishes the shares that would otherwise belong to more industrious, and more worthy members; and thus in the same manner forces more to become dependent.[52]

This assault was in the first edition of his *Essay* and reiterated at length in subsequent editions. Just like Pitt's Poor Bill, socially sanctioned 'philanthropic' institutions threatened the mainsprings of population by encouraging vice and turning a blind eye to moral responsibilities. They operated under illusions of life and liberty that they could not possibly realise, a criticism that voluntary charity nominally evaded since their selectivity meant the poor could not grow dependent upon them.[53] The best prospects for the future were in committed labour that sought to increase means of subsistence. As Malthus concluded, if the government endeavoured to 'encourage and direct the industry of the farmers, and circulate the best information on agricultural subjects, it would do much more for the population of the country than by the establishment of five hundred foundling hospitals'.[54]

Conclusion: the Critics

Malthus's Scandinavian tour was on the one hand designed as a fact-finding mission to help him overcome his critics' objections that the first *Essay* was too theoretical and 'inapplicable to the present state of society'. But his observations, data, and personal interviews were woven into the narrative of the second edition to create a scientific argument that made his revised argument resemble a travelogue more than a theoretical treatise. The condition of Europe was viewed relative to the effects of his 'law of human nature'. His comparisons of health, work-regimes, climate, agrarian cultivation, and government administration within Scandinavia, and between the northern with other European countries, helped him hone his illustrations of preventative versus positive checks to population growth.

So how accurate was he? Some contemporary critics objected to his assault on charity, others to his presumption that 'laws of human nature' rather than divine ordinance govern the health of the population. Christian apologists rejected the empirical data about trends in population growth and protested from the pulpit that he contradicted the Bible and denied providence. Puritan pamphleteers accused him of atheism.[55] For most, it was easy to attack his conclusions rather than his 'facts' or premises. Many conceded that the evidence proved that population does have a tendency to expand, but, in Godwin's words, claimed that Malthus underestimated the 'resources of the human mind' in coping with these problems.[56] Arthur Young, who expressed his own fears of population growth in his *Travels in France*, condemned Malthus's refusal of relief for the poor and proposed a remedy of offering potato plots to labourers to look after themselves.[57] The philosophising poet Samuel Coleridge found fault with Malthus's line of reasoning, and declared that his argument amounted to little more than an 'entertaining farrago of quotations from books of travels, &c'.[58] Even Clarke, Malthus's part-time travelling companion, had different views than Malthus. Clarke's views were more encouraging of the Swedish government's interest in, and patronage of, science and medicine – in establishing institutional and educational programmes, for example.[59]

Other reviewers were more receptive of Malthus's doctrine, and were embraced by the bulk of politicians, economists, and the public. A reviewer in *The Monthly Review* agreed that commerce and manufacturers had grown to be appendages too predominate in the national economy, and was sympathetic to his warnings about over-reliance on medical policy, linking diseased human and political bodies: 'the body politic is in an artificial, and in some degree, diseased state, with one of its principal members out of proportion to the rest. Almost all medicine is in itself bad; and one of the great evils of illness is, the necessity of taking it. No person can well be more averse to medicine in the animal economy, or a system of expedients in political economy, than myself ....'[60] With the exception of Christian apologists, few seem to have criticised Malthus's use of empirical 'facts' about the rates of population growth and his observations about checks to population abroad. The 'cases' of Norway, Sweden, Russia, as well as France and Switzerland (where he visited during the Peace of Amiens in 1802), were referred to by some reviewers as the obviously unproblematic proofs used in support of his conclusions. As Francis Jeffrey in the *Edinburgh Review* sympathetically opined, it was 'for having stated, with inimitable caution and accuracy, facts which cannot possibly be called into question, that Mr Malthus has been accused of sophistry, of presumption, of blasphemy, inhumanity and love of vice and corruption'.[61] Among Malthus's many converts, he could boast Pitt, Paley, James Mill, Nassau Senior, Henry Brougham, Thomas Chalmers, David Ricardo, and, famously, Charles Darwin.[62]

Modern scholars have grown more sceptical. In the last fifty years or so, Swedish demographers have re-examined the eighteenth-century statistics and reconsidered the accuracy and uses of the Malthusian model to interpret population trends.[63] Eli Heckscher, in a 1943 article, claimed that the mortality rate in Norway was slightly higher than what Malthus determined, about 25 rather than 20.8 per 1000. He also suggested that the differences between Norway and Sweden were not as great as Malthus claimed, but that the Scandinavian countries as a whole showed a marked contrast to other European states. Gustaf Utterström is critical of Heckscher's (and Malthus's) suggestion that harvest fluctuations were the main factor underlying mortality in the pre 1820 period. He emphasises epidemics, climate, poor housing, and hygiene. Malthus suggested that certain factors in Norwegian agrarian lifestyles – parish control, property and inheritance rights, and other less apparent local 'customs' – resulted in the reinforcement of 'moral restraint' which became the strongest preventative check to population. He warned against the Swedish model, accusing their system that unnecessarily provides, *gratis*, support for the ailing. The collaboration between the *Collegium Medicum* and the Swedish Parliament wasted funds that could be better spent on creating agricultural work. Twentieth-century scholars re-evaluating the constraints to population growth in Scandinavia have proposed their own notions of 'homeo-static equilibriums' and 'local human ecological situations' to help interpret the balance between natural resources and population. What emerges is not a general judgement about the 'validity' of Malthus's arguments regarding Scandinavia, but competing particular conclusions. While some economic theorists still purport to be Malthusian in character, my concern here has been more with Malthus's own accounts and presentation of evidence, and the ways that his experiences abroad – of health care, mortality rates, marriage practices, and so on, informed the significantly rewritten second and subsequent editions of his *Essay*.

Notes

1. Karin Johannisson, 'Society in Numbers: The Debate over Quantification in 18th-Century Political Economy', in Tore Frängsmyr, J.L. Heilbron, and Robin Rider (eds), *The Quantifying Spirit in the 18th Century* (Berkeley and Oxford: University of California Press, 1990), 343–61; Roger Smith, *The Fontana History of the Human Sciences* (London: Fontana, 1997), 313–14.
2. Gerd Gigerenzer, Zeno Swijtink, Theodore Porter, Lorraine Daston, John Beatty, Lorenz Krüger, *The Empire of Chance: How Probability Changed Science and Everyday Life* (Cambridge: Cambridge University Press, 1989).
3. E. Arosenius, 'The History and Organization of Swedish Official Statistics', in John Koren (ed.), *The History of Statistics* (New York: American Statistical Association, 1918).
4. W. Coxe, *Travels into Poland, Russia, Sweden...* (London, 1784), iii, 380–85; E. D. Clarke, *Travels in Various Countries of Europe*, 11 vols (London, 1816–24), xi, 147.
5. Keith Michael Baker, *Condorcet: From Natural Philosophy to Social Mathematics* (1975, 1982).
6. Thomas Robert Malthus, *An Essay on the Principle of Population, as it Affects the Future Improvement of Society, with Remarks on the Speculations of Mr. Godwin, M. Condorcet, and Other Writers* (London: J. Johnson, 1798; facsimile reprint, Macmillan, 1966), 165–9.
7. Malthus, *Essay* (1798), 193; see John Avery, *Progress, Poverty, and Population: Re-reading Condorcet, Godwin, and Malthus* (Essex: Frank Cass, 1997), for renewed general account of the different ways these writers tackled population problems and addressed issues of progress and human happiness.
8. Malthus, *Essay* (1798), 62–3 for preventative checks amongst the 'lower classes'.
9. Malthus, *Essay* (1798), 395; for natural theology and Christian demography, see Boyd Hilton, *The Age of Atonement: The Influence of Evangelicalism on Social and Economic Thought* (Oxford: Clarendon Press, 1988), especially chapter three; also Gigerenzer, *et al.*, *The Empire of Chance*, chapter one for Süssmilch; James Bonar, *Malthus and His Work* (London: Frank Cass, 1885; 1966), 34–5 for Paley.
10. Quoted in Bonar, *Malthus*, 49; see also his chapter on the critics, 355–99.
11. Thomas Robert Malthus, *An Investigation of the Cause of the Present High Price of Provisions* (London: J. Johnson, 1800), 28.
12. Richard Price, *Observations on Reversionary Payments* (first edn,

London, 1771); Ian Hacking, *The Taming of Chance* (Cambridge: Cambridge University Press, 1990), 49–51.

13. For Süssmilch's *Die göttliche Ordnung in den Veränderungen des menschlichen Geschlechts, aus der Geburt, dem Tode und der Fortpflanzung desselben erwiesen* (first edn, 1741) (*God's Plan for the Development of the Human Race, as Demonstrated by the Births, Deaths and Propagation of the Same*), see Gigerenzer, *et al., The Empire of Chance*, 40; Hacking, *Taming of Chance*, 40; for Malthus's familiarity of Süssmilch's work, see James, *Population Malthus*. As in the first edition, Malthus, in the second edition, comments on the kind of minute attention to the manners and customs of the 'lower classes of society' that is necessary to draw accurate inferences upon the causes of the checks to population. Malthus was happy to acknowledge that 'This branch of statistical knowledge has of late years been attended to in some countries'. In particular, he drew attention to 'the judicious questions which Sir John Sinclair circulated in Scotland, and the very valuable accounts which he has collected in that part of the island .... If, with a few subordinate improvements, this work had contained accurate and complete registers for the last 150 years, it would have been inestimable, and would have exhibited a better picture of the internal state of a country, than has yet been presented to the world'. The reference to Sinclair, President of the Board of Agriculture (1793–98 and 1806–13), relates to the 160 questions he sent to ministers of the Church of Scotland regarding parish soils, climate, diseases, births, deaths, marriages, rents, and other topics on the environment and social customs. The answers were published between 1791 and 1799 in *The Statistical Account of Scotland*, 21 volumes. While these statistics reflected only ten, rather than the obviously preferred '150 years', Malthus nonetheless was also able to refer to Sweden's 50-year-old statistical registers, which did present the best picture of the internal state of the country; *Essay* (1803), I, 21–2.

14. Malthus, *Essay* (1803), 58.

15. For general discussion of uses of travel literature, see Brian Dolan, *Exploring European Frontiers: British Travellers in the Age of Enlightenment* (Basingstoke: Macmillan, 2000).

16. Malthus, *Essay* (1803), 148, emphasis added.

17. Malthus's Norwegian diaries are still extant and have been published as Patricia James (ed.), *The Travel Diaries of T.R. Malthus* (Cambridge: Cambridge University Press, 1966); his other diaries, covering Sweden and Russia, were lost after he lent them to Clarke, who used them to help write his own *Travels*.

18. Malthus, *Travel Diaries*, 208; Malthus, *Essay* (1803), 148.

19. Quoted from Johannisson, 'Why Cure the Sick? Population Policy and Health Programs within 18th-Century Swedish Mercantilism', in Anders Brändström and Lars-Göran Tedebrand (eds), *Society, Health and Population during the Demographic Transition* (Stockholm: Almqvist and Wiksell, 1988), 323–30, on 325.

20. Malthus, *Essay* (1803), 72; [Thomas Short], *A General Chronological History of the Air, Weather, Seasons, Meteors, &c. in Sundry Places and Different Times; More Particularly for the Space of 250 Years, Together with some of their most Remarkable Effects on Animal (especially Human) Bodies and Vegetables*, 2 vols (London, 1749).

21. Malthus, *Travel Diaries*, 202; in his *Essay* (1803), he noted that boys who drive the plough looked older and were more robust than their counterparts in countries elsewhere on the continent, 153; compare with earlier thoughts on physical appearance and labour in *Essay* (1798), 73.

22. Pontoppidan, *Natural History of Norway*, 245, quoted in Malthus, *Travel Diaries*, 145.

23. Malthus, *Travel Diaries*, 175.

24. David Cannadine, 'Conspicuous Consumption by the Landed Classes, 1790-1830', in Michael Turner (ed.), *Malthus and His Time* (London: Macmillan, 1986), 96-111.

25. Malthus, *Essay* (1803), 134, referring to David Hume's *On Population*, 1768, 467.

26. See D. Harvey, 'Population, Resources, and the Ideology of Science', in John C. Wood (ed.), *Thomas Robert Malthus: Critical Assessments*, 4 vols (London: Croom Helm, 1986) i, 308–35, Smith on 314.

27. Keith Tribe, *Land, Labour, and Economic Discourse* (London: Routledge and Kegan Paul, 1978), chapter five.

28. Malthus, *Essay* (1803), 153.

29. See also Malthus's qualifying remarks on manufactures in his *Observations on the Effects of the Corn Laws* (London, 1814), 71. For the different types of manufacturer and relationship between agriculture and industry, see Maxine Berg, *The Age of Manufacturers: Industry, Innovation and Work in Britain, 1700-1820* (London: Basil Blackwell, 1985).

30. Although Norway was devoid of plague and extensive losses from war, Malthus seems to have been ignorant of, or too easily overlooked, the years of famine and epidemics that are reflected in Norwegian population statistics.

31. Malthus, *Travel Diaries*, 89.

32. Malthus, *Essay* (1803), 150.

33. Malthus, *Essay* (1803), 150.
34. Malthus, *Essay* (1803), 18, for introduction and definition of term.
35. For discussion of this, see James Bonar's notes to the first *Essay* (Macmillan, 1966), xx.
36. On the correlation between population increases and early marriages, see E.A. Wrigley and R.S. Schofield, *The Population History of England 1541-1871: A Reconstruction* (new edition, Cambridge: Cambridge University Press, 1989).
37. Malthus, *Essay* (1803), 157.
38. Malthus, *Essay* (1803), 158.
39. Malthus, *Essay* (1803), 153.
40. Malthus, *Essay* (1803), 159.
41. Karin Johannisson, 'Why cure the sick?'.
42. Phrase used by Charles Rosen to describe statistics on population and health; for general discussion, see his *A History of Public Health* (New York, 1958, new edition: Johns Hopkins, 1993), 148–52; for revised history of population health, including an account of eighteenth-century Sweden, see Dorothy Porter, *Health, Civilisation, and the State: A History of Public Health from Antiquity to Modernity* (London: Routledge, 1999).
43. Malthus's travel diaries for the Swedish leg of his Scandinavian tour was lost after he lent them to Edward Daniel Clarke, but the biographical register to Patricia James's edition of the *Essay* are useful.
44. Salim Rashid, 'Malthus's *Essay on Population*: The Facts of 'Super-Growth' and the Rhetoric of Scientific Persuasion', *Journal for the History of Behavioural Sciences* 23 (1987), 22–36, for the credibility of Malthus's 'facts'; Patricia James's notes to the second edition of Malthus's *Essay* points out citation errors and discusses alternatives to blatant distortions; for Malthus's disclaimer, see his preface to the second edition.
45. Malthus, *Essay* (1803), 162.
46. Eva Nyström, 'The Development of Cause-of-Death Classification in Eighteenth Century Sweden: A Survey of Problems, Sources, and Possibilities', in Brändström and Tedebrand (eds), *Society, Health, and Population*, 109–30.
47. Dorothy Porter, 'Public Health', in W. Bynum and Roy Porter (eds), *Companion Encyclopaedia of the History of Medicine*, 2 vols (London: Routledge, 1993) ii, 1231–1261.
48. Johannisson, 'The People's Health: Public Health Policies in Sweden', in Dorothy Porter (ed.), *The History of Public Health and the Modern State* (Amsterdam: Rodopi, 1994), 165-182, on 168.

49. *Ibid*, 167.

50. Malthus, *Essay* (1803), 164-165.

51. Malthus, *Essay* (1803), 176, in his chapter on Russia, where he also travelled during his northern tour.

52. Malthus, *Essay* (1798), 83-84.

53. Anne Digby, 'Malthus and the Reform of the English Poor Law', in Michael Turner (ed.), *Malthus and His Time*, 157–69.

54. Malthus, *Essay* (1803), 164; in 1826 Malthus added to this conclusion an observation that, since the introduction of vaccination to Sweden in 1804 and due to the progress of agriculture and industry, the healthiness and population of the country had considerably advanced.

55. Hawick, 1807, 'A Sumons of Wakening'; Bonar, *Malthus and his Work*, 365.

56. Bonar, *Malthus and his Work*, 360.

57. Digby, 'Malthus and the Reform'.

58. His manuscript comments in his copy of Malthus's second edition quoted in Bonar, *Malthus and his Work*, 375.

59. However, Clarke's testimony that the population in southern European countries seems to have grown to push the limits of its supply was invoked in support of Malthus by some reviewers: see Pyle (ed.), *Population*, 262.

60. *The Monthly Review*, xlii (December, 1803), quotted in Andrew Pyle (ed.), *Population: Contemporary Responses to Thomas Malthus* (Bristol: Thoemmes Press, 1994), 54.

61. [Francis Jeffrey] in reply to Malthus's critics, in the *Edinburgh Review* (August 1810), quoted in Pyle (ed.), *Population*, 212; see also Bernard Semmel (ed.), *Occasional Papers of T.R. Malthus on Ireland, Population, and Political Economy* (New York: Burt Franklin, 1963), 269-281.

62. See Hilton, *Age of Atonement*, for contemporary economic responses to Malthus.

63. For discussion of the following articles, see Lars Magnusson, 'Malthus in Scandinavia, 1799', in Turner (ed.), *Malthus and His Time*, 60-70.

2

Boys to Men:
Moral Restraint at Haileybury College

Timothy L. Alborn

Britain in the early nineteenth century has been variously described as an age of atonement and as poised between two overlapping ages of empire.[1] Both themes, furthermore, have a direct bearing on the place of the City of London in British politics and culture at that time. Boyd Hilton has shown how the ideas of atonement and moral restraint were far from irrelevant to City men who worried about the speculative propensities of the age; and the City as a focal point for empire has long been a staple of imperial historiography. Like coaches in the London fog, however, these two themes often cross paths in studies of the City without acknowledging each others' presence. One person whose career straddles both themes is Thomas Robert Malthus, whose seminal advocacy of moral restraint in social relations makes him a key figure in studies like Hilton's, and whose two decades of service working for the East India Company (a notorious bastion of City power) gave him a chance to extend his famous moral views into the arena of Empire.

This chapter seeks to establish a common context for the themes of atonement, empire and the City by analysing the formation and reception of Malthus's *Statements Regarding the East-India College* (1817). On the surface, this pamphlet was little more than a hastily-composed defence of Haileybury College, where he taught future company servants, against charges from shareholders and politicians that students there were undisciplined and poorly educated. But upon closer scrutiny the pamphlet reveals two sides to Malthus's career, moral restraint and empire, that met in a revealing dialogue with East India shareholders over the all-too-lively bodies of his adolescent students. One obvious focus of moral restraint in the pamphlet was the students themselves, whom Malthus hoped to teach how to act like adults so they could fend off the amplified temptations that would await them in India. But Malthus also claimed that Haileybury was useful for restraining the corrosive effects of patronage that had long been a problem among company shareholders. He pointed out that the college forced parents to think twice about securing Indian appointments for manifestly incompetent relatives, by interposing the risk that patrons' nominees who failed to pass muster might be expelled from the college before ever making it to India.

In addition to shedding new light on Malthus's conception of moral restraint, his East India pamphlet also revealed contradictions inhering in that conception, which have been discussed in the context of his population theory.[2] Regarding population, Malthus confronted the dilemma that the healthy (and godly) activity of reproduction by married adults tended to produce the unhealthy social consequence of overpopulation. After first presenting the problem in the stark terms of 'positive' checks like famine and disease in the first edition of his *Essay on the Principle of Population* (1798), he later adopted a more optimistic view that included a role for consumerism as a means of suppressing the more primal instincts of the poor. By 1817, he was ready to assert that as emerging market institutions intruded into more people's lives, goods that had once been regarded as luxuries would now be deemed necessaries of life. He hoped that this development, in turn, would induce the sort of moral restraint among the lower classes that he had only imputed to the 'middle orders' in his earlier writings.[3] But try as he might to contain moral restraint within the 'natural' realm of economic laws, he and his successors were ultimately faced with a stark choice between coercively restraining the human propensity to breed – relying on such makeshifts as the new poor law to provide preventive checks where the market had failed – or standing by as 'positive' checks to population growth took hold. His commitment to moral restraint as a preferable solution to the problem of overpopulation, in short, begged the question of who should do the restraining.

Malthus faced a similar dilemma (if not as global) when he applied his ideas about moral restraint to the case of the East India Company. As in the economy at large, where he hoped a developing set of market institutions would uncoercively restrain early marriages, he hoped the establishment of Haileybury College would provide a spontaneous economic incentive for company shareholders to restrain their own desire for patronage. Extra costs like tuition and the risk of expulsion, which had previously been viewed as luxuries, would come to be seen as a necessary prelude to life in East India, just as tuition at Oxford or Cambridge had become a 'necessary luxury' for elites who hoped to secure ecclesiastical posts for their children.

These strictly economic incentives, Malthus hoped, would keep shareholders' desire for patronage from interfering with the teaching staff's disciplinary efforts. As in the more general case, however, 'natural' economic laws were inadequate to the task of providing Malthus's hoped-for balance between self-restraint and commercial prosperity. This inadequacy, which in the realm of social reform expressed itself in recurrent appeals to government intervention, resulted in the Indian case in a choice between continued abuses of patronage (paired with continued disciplinary problems at Haileybury) and a more bureaucratic solution to civil service reform. When reformers finally turned to the latter solution, they replaced the private company with the public India Office, and replaced patronage with state-administered competitive examinations of incoming students.

The question of patronage was intimately connected with the issue of which set of people controlled the minds and bodies of the late-teens who were being trained for service in India. Malthus was convinced that his students' parents, many of whom were shareholders with a powerful electoral and financial stake in the company, had far too much ability to blunt disciplinary efforts at Haileybury by getting the company's directors to reverse the professors' decisions. He charged that discipline at Haileybury suffered when parents openly criticised Haileybury or pampered their children. Parents, for their part, blamed disciplinary lapses on the professors' failure to maintain authority over their students. Instead of waiting for riots to happen and then singling out the ringleaders for expulsion, they argued, Malthus and his fellow professors needed to work harder to generate respect among students before things got out of hand.

Underpinning this debate about who should wield power over the student body was a deeper controversy over the maturation process of Haileybury pupils as they grew from boys into men. When these students arrived in Hertfordshire at the age of sixteen, they encountered a *college* environment which their public-school counterparts would not experience for several more years: caps and gowns, 'professors' (not tutors) who gave lectures instead of lessons, and a system of discipline which abjured corporal punishment and allowed far more free time than was the case at other public schools. All this accorded with Malthus's goal of inoculating his students with a taste of the liberties that he assumed they would face in India. But one result of this early exposure to freedom, in the eyes of many critics, was an abnormal incidence of delinquency, which in turn resulted in the painful recourse to expulsion. In defending

Haileybury's collegiate structure, Malthus offered a very different interpretation of its high levels of delinquency and consequent expulsion. As in his more general conception of moral restraint, he was happy to accept some (duly punished) bad behaviour, provided that the punishment taught others to restrain their own desires. Expulsion, in this setting, served the dual purpose of showing existing students the consequences of their actions and devaluing the currency of patronage in the eyes of would-be company shareholders. Malthus was more than willing to live with these relatively innocuous wages of sin, in order to stave off the more deadly consequences of bad behaviour among undisciplined company men in India.

Corrupt Constitutions:
Adam Smith and Edmund Burke on India

Malthus's assumption that economic incentives could compel moral restraint echoed Adam Smith's observations in *The Wealth of Nations* about the disciplinary effect of market forces. Unlike Malthus, however, who ambitiously (and problematically) tried to extend the idea of market discipline in such institutional settings as the East India Company and poor law reform, Smith drew a line between individual enterprise, where the market exerted constructive discipline, and institutions, where unhindered market forces always carried the threat of corruption. As did most eighteenth-century political theorists, Smith assumed that whatever discipline was to be had in the political realm would need to come from a natural aristocracy – a set of disinterested rulers who were oblivious to the corrupting effects of self-interested seekers of patronage and mercantilist economic policies. When he applied this idea to workings of the state, Smith assumed that corruption of the natural aristocracy was most likely to cause problems in the case of mercantilism, which threatened to derail economic growth. He viewed patronage in Parliament as unfortunate, but not in itself capable of preventing the free market from creating growth; patronage also had the advantage of providing certain key legislators with the requisite power to create a 'system of management' that Smith felt was necessary for maintaining the 'civil and military establishment' of the country.[4]

Smith was more concerned about the corrupting powers of patronage in the East India Company, since it combined the commercial function of foreign trade with the political function of governing the Indian natives. Part of his concern was due to the company's hybrid character, which had led its servants to view their legislative duties as 'but an appendix to that of the merchant'. The grasping nature of company employees (combined with the powerlessness of the native Indians to resist them) led to the anomalous result that civil servants in India had the potential of making more money from their positions than shareholders could earn in dividends. And this situation, in turn, gave shareholders an incentive to encourage corruption among servants, by pressuring the directors to hire their relatives for such positions instead of clamping down on corruption in the name of administrative efficiency. In most firms, shareholders paid little attention to the servants hired by their directors, apart from possibly expressing concern about high salaries cutting into their profits. But in the East India Company a whole class of proprietors had evolved who hoped to gain indirectly from the short-term profits that accrued to local servants. With little regard for the effect of their actions on their own relatively insubstantial dividend, these proprietors paid in their £1400 for 'a share, though not in the plunder, yet in the appointment of the plunderers of India'.[5]

To this strictly economic argument against patronage, Smith's friend Edmund Burke added a sexual variant to the threat of Indian corruption. Burke, who together with Charles Fox led the late-eighteenth century Parliamentary battle against the East India Company, made an impassioned plea to protect the Indian natives from the firm's youthful soldiers and tax collectors who 'drink the intoxicating draught of authority and dominion before their heads are able to bear it'. A political body corrupted by greedy shareholders, he worried, would translate directly into corrupt physical bodies among the company's servants – which in turn would infect the purity of the ageless Indian system of ranks. In his speech on Fox's East India Bill in 1783, Burke envisioned 'wave after wave' of '[y]oung men (boys almost)' rolling into India, 'with appetites continually renewing for a food that is constantly wasting'. To reinforce his point that these youths were being *corrupted* by their early exposure to India, and were not innately immoral, he added that there was 'nothing in the boys we send to India worse than in the boys whom we are whipping at school'; the problem was that in India, 'neither Nature nor reason have any opportunity to exert themselves for remedy of the excesses of their premature power'.[6]

Neither Smith's appeal to conflicting economic motives nor Burke's more dramatic appeal to sexual excess, however, succeeded in transferring patronage from the company to what they both agreed was the safer refuge of a government ministry. In 1783, when Burke and Fox called for Indian affairs to be handed over to a government board with a term of four years, they met with strenuous criticism from opposing politicians who assumed they intended to build on the patronage opportunities such a board would give them to make future opposition impossible. Although Fox's opponents failed to defeat his bill in Commons, they convinced George III to secure its defeat in Lords and to call for a new election, in which Fox's supporters were voted out of power by an electorate who feared for their constitutional liberties. William Pitt and Henry Dundas, who took office upon the 1784 election, avoided the pitfall of transferring patronage to the Crown in their India Bill, which installed the Board of Control that would supervise the company for the next seven decades.[7]

In the half-century following Pitt's India Bill, company apologists met the charge of patronage in one of two ways.[8] Their first defence was simply to present company patronage as the lesser of two evils, with the greater evil being the dispensation of Indian patronage by a minister of state. This response succeeded in preserving the status quo, since both Parliament and George III were deeply suspicious of ministerial power, but it did not offer a constructive solution to the problems of plunder in India and jobbery at home. A more constructive response, initiated by Lord Wellesley during his tenure as Governor General and seconded by Malthus at Haileybury, pointed to an improved system of education within the company. According to this plan, which was in fact consistent with Smith's general views on education, the right sort of training (together with other administrative reforms introduced by the Board of Control) would diminish the 'plundering' proclivities of company servants.[9]

Pitt's successful appeal to the greater evil of ministerial patronage had stymied the Smithian critique of 'plunderers' and their patrons without really answering it. When company officials did act more constructively towards improving the situation, it was at the prodding of Lord Wellesley in his capacity as Governor General, who in 1800 established a college in Calcutta. The directors, despite soon closing the college against the wishes of Wellesley and the Board of Control, eventually did respond to his implicit critique of their existing methods of selecting and training officials by founding Haileybury College in Hertfordshire six years later. Simply establishing Haileybury did not directly address either the problem of plunder in India or the shareholders' role in appointing the plunderers, since the directors retained final authority over determining which college graduates were fit to be shipped abroad. Throughout much of its duration, Haileybury only signified to shareholders another hurdle (and for many, an especially onerous one) which they needed to cross in order to make a case to directors on behalf of a friend or relative.[10]

The chief focus of shareholder resistance to Haileybury was its self-styled identity as a 'college' for students in their late teens, whose upper-class counterparts were still nearing the end of their education at schools like Harrow and Charterhouse. In order to prepare students for their special responsibilities in India, Haileybury spurned the public school regimen of corporal punishment and rote lessons in favour of a system in which students wore caps and gowns and attended lectures on Sanskrit and political economy. To critics, such a system recreated in England the same problem that Burke had complained of in India, where youths were prematurely thrust into a situation in which their uncontrolled adolescent desires held full sway. New arrivals at Haileybury, complained one shareholder in 1811, were 'liberated from the salutary bondage of mental constraint' which they had endured at public school, and were treated to the 'dangerous delusion, that they have arrived at a premature manhood'. If Haileybury students were subject to this delusion, so too were their 'professors', who sought, 'by foolish titles, to impose an idea that they are something more than school-masters'. Whatever justification there might be for treating teenagers as if they were men, this did not alter the fact that they were still boys, as the shareholder's caustic conclusion made clear: 'if we can convey this rapid growth to their minds, we can, no doubt, do the same to their bodies: – let us put them into man's attire, and bid their limbs and sinews expand till they fill their clothes'.[11]

This type of complaint appeared especially frequently on the many occasions between 1809 and 1817 in which Haileybury was rocked by rioting and other forms of delinquency. Disturbances in 1809 led the entire student body to be temporarily 'rusticated'; two years later nearly forty students were disciplined for 'tumultuously assembling' for five days to protest 'bad dinners' and being deprived of pistols on Guy Fawkes Day. Following a period of relative quiet, even more violent behaviour surfaced in November 1815 when a group of fourteen students wearing fencing masks physically assaulted the college's steward and his assistant. In response, the company paid for the victims to bring charges before the Hertford Magistrate, resulting in a brief prison stay for three of the boys (to await trial with a possible verdict of hanging) and more negative publicity for the college.[12] The incident produced an alarming twist on Haileybury's mission of treating teenagers as if they were men: in urging the company to bring the 1815 assault before the magistrate, the shareholder Francis Horner observed that 'if you cannot punish your pupils as boys, you must subject them to the punishments by which other men are kept in order'.[13]

Malthus's *Statements*: Turning boys into men

Malthus first defended his college for boys in 1813, in response to the disturbance in 1811, and again in 1817 after the attack on the staff members led a group of company shareholders to call for Haileybury to be abolished. In pamphlets published at these times, he invoked Smith's concern, as expressed by Wellesley in 1800, that Indian civil servants needed to behave as 'ministers and officers of a *powerful sovereign*' and not as 'the agents of a *commercial concern*'. By following the lead of Wellesley's original proposal for Fort William, however, Malthus departed from Smith's assumption that company officials could never be taught how to act like statesmen. All that was needed, he claimed, was 'to give them a superior education': this would be sufficient to answer '[o]ne of the great objections urged by Adam Smith against the government of an exclusive Company' by ensuring that 'the feelings of the sovereign conspicuously predominated' over those of the merchant.[14] He further insisted that a crucial element in this 'superior education' was Haileybury's collegiate structure, which taught candidates for Indian service lessons that could never be transmitted in a mere school. On this point, he was especially concerned to dispute the charge that Haileybury was simply an English version of the cesspool of indiscipline that Burke had discerned in India. Instead, he claimed, it was exactly because such dangers awaited young men abroad that some prior exposure to the 'liberties' of adulthood was necessary, and he reasoned that it was far better to provide that exposure in Haileybury than in Calcutta.

In forming his defence of Haileybury, Malthus borrowed freely from the creed of moral restraint that he was busy developing when not teaching future nabobs. In the much-expanded 1803 edition of the *Essay on the Principle of Population*, published two years before he started teaching at the college, Malthus developed his concept of moral restraint in order 'to soften some of the harshest conclusions' of the 1798 edition, in which he had predicted that population pressure would lead to a stagnant economy punctuated by bouts of famine and plague.[15] Though more optimistic, the new edition of the *Essay* still relied on the palpable presence of 'positive checks', which were evident in much of the contemporary world as well as in England's recent past, to convince people that postponement of marriage was a far preferable solution to the problem of overpopulation. Malthus followed William Paley in assuming that moral lessons would only be effective if they were confirmed by experience. And if, as he claimed in the *Essay*, 'a strict attention to... consequences, and the regulation of our conduct conformably to them' was 'our principal duty', then a continued insistence on the effects of unrestrained sexual desire was surely necessary from a moral standpoint.[16]

An important feature in Malthus's emerging defence of moral restraint was the disciplinary potential of the market to temper people's more basic sexual urges. By 1806, a year after accepting the post at Haileybury, he was ready to admit in the third edition of the *Essay* that 'manufactures, by inspiring a taste for comforts, tend to promote a favourable change' in the 'permanent habits' of the working poor. And in 1817, the same year he published his defence of the college, a new edition of the *Essay* proclaimed that the consumption of luxury goods tended 'unquestionably to improve the mind and elevate the character'.[17] By stressing the positive (and morally elevating) allurements of luxuries in this way, Malthus further softened the process by which population pressure would be averted. If in 1803 he claimed that people could exercise moral restraint, but only by constantly brooding on the harsh consequences of failing to do so, by 1817 he was willing to intersperse these periods of self-examination with the more pleasurable diversions of the market. Although all these passages were specifically directed at working people, they in fact had much bearing on the situation at Haileybury, since both issues pointed to *education* as the key to achieving 'personal responsibility'.[18]

Malthus's prophylactic appeal to moral restraint, combined with his newly optimistic regard for the 'elevated' pleasures of consumption, resurfaced when he moved from English paupers to Haileybury pupils. The relatively old age at which children entered Haileybury suggested to their teacher a capacity 'to be influenced by the higher motives of the love of distinction and the fear of disgrace' – a more constructive sort of motivation than 'being kept to their studies solely by the fear of immediate observation and punishment'. As with other forms of consumption, which were always about *choosing* between higher and lower forms of pleasure, the perquisites of collegiate life would lead to moral restraint only if the student acquired a taste for them of his own free will. Hence each student was given 'the opportunity of choosing his own society' while at Haileybury and was taught 'the habit of regulating his own time'.

This came in the form of 'a separate room' for each student (as opposed to a bed in a dormitory), in which 'he breakfasts, drinks tea, and prepares his lectures'. Malthus viewed these unsupervised intervals as a character-building exercise, in which students would learn 'to conduct themselves in a situation in which they are subjected to no discipline'. Only in this way would it be possible to achieve Haileybury's 'specific object', which was 'to inculcate, gradually, manly feelings, manly studies, and manly self-controul, rather earlier than usual' – on the grounds that '[t]hose who go out to India, must and will be men the moment they reach the country... and there they will be immediately exposed to temptations of no common magnitude and danger'.[19]

By reframing the problem of discipline in India in terms of moral restraint, Malthus was self-consciously building on arguments developed by Smith and Burke. His most direct debt to Smith concerned his conviction that Indian servants needed to be taught how to be statesmen, not tradesmen. This was clear in his response to the company director Randall Jackson, who in 1815 had attacked Haileybury's collegiate pretensions on the grounds that such conditions were not needed to teach boys how to 'weigh tea, count bales, and measure muslins'. Malthus replied with a long list of company posts which were 'quite unconnected with trade', involving jurisprudence, taxation, and diplomacy, and which added up to 400 out of the 472 assignments which were periodically open to Haileybury graduates.[20] At a deeper level, he also defended Haileybury in terms that indicate the influence of Smith's *Theory of Moral Sentiments*, which presented emulation as the most important factor in motivating human behaviour.[21] Malthus used similar moral arguments to defend the granting of 'medals, prizes of books, and honorary distinctions' to students as a means of 'exciting emulation and industry'. Here he was also rehearsing his idea that 'permanent habits' of restraint could best be achieved by the diversionary lure of 'elevating' luxuries. The 'new stimulants' on offer to students in Haileybury's lecture halls and prize competitions, he concluded, 'had wrought a most beneficial change in their feelings and habits'.[22]

Malthus's application of moral restraint to Haileybury also built on Edmund Burke's sensational account of the unruly exploits of English adolescents in India. He clearly bought into Burke's stereotype of India as a seedbed of vice in the 1803 edition of the *Essay*, where he presented India as a country in which a surplus of food led people 'to prefer the luxury of idleness to the luxury of improved lodging and clothing'.[23] He repeated these assumptions in his pamphlet on

Haileybury, citing 'the seductions' of India's 'luxurious climate' and worrying that a teenager in India would be 'surrounded by natives devoted to his will' and 'tempted to indulgences of all kinds by the novel forms in which they present themselves'. Such concerns, in the context of his high hopes for the 'new stimulants' at Haileybury, clearly indicate that he only counted some forms of consumption as likely to inculcate habits of moral restraint. The advantage of the college, in this regard, was that it controlled the flow of goods and services without interfering with students' ability to choose whether or not to partake of them. Turning boys into men meant teaching boys the proper way to consume.[24]

Malthus similarly appealed to moral restraint to defend the practice of removing pupils who failed to act like adults when given the chance. Expelling an unruly student while he was still in England would prevent the more serious consequences that would follow from shipping libertines to India. It 'cannot surely be a matter of regret', he urged, 'that those who have shewn headstrong, refractory, and capricious tempers... should not be allowed to go out to India, and be furnished with an opportunity of tryannising over its suffering inhabitants'. The only losers in this case were the students themselves – and sacrificing the occasional student on the altar of discipline had the salutary effect of bringing home 'the fear of disgrace' to other students in no uncertain terms. The occasional outbreak of rioting in the controlled environs of Haileybury, followed by swift punishment, would effectively restrain the behaviour of the remaining students, and teach them a lesson that would continue to regulate their actions abroad. Expulsion, concluded Malthus, was 'a painful, but necessary, sacrifice to those general rules, the gross violation of which cannot be passed over without a sacrifice of much greater and more general interests'.[25]

Many shareholders and other critics of Haileybury refused to accept this line of reasoning, claiming instead that rioting at the college signified a failure by the staff and the system to work properly. The *Times*, which Malthus had singled out in his pamphlet for its prior attacks on Haileybury's collegiate pretensions, once again led the attack when his pamphlet appeared in 1817 – insisting that

> the application of... an hyper-collegiate system to the management
> and instruction of boys from the beginning of 16 to 18 years of age,
> is improper; and that caps and gowns, Messieurs the Professors, and
> a Mr. Principal, are all calculated to instil and diffuse an illusion, that
> the students are and ought to be free from restraint at an age when

they are not qualified to govern themselves.

As in 1811, critics claimed that it was wishful thinking to expect boys to act like anything other than boys, regardless of the environment into which they were placed. Indeed, Malthus's famous anti-perfectionism meant that he was an especially rich target for such complaints, as when the shareholder Douglas Kinnaird chastised Malthus's 'Utopia of education' at Haileybury.[26]

In casting Malthus in the role that had been reserved for Godwin and Condorcet in the *Essay on Population*, Kinnaird ignored Malthus's basic assumption that not all children would be able to survive Haileybury without succumbing to the temptation to riot; and that those children, if Malthus had his way, would be summarily expelled for their weakness. This failure (or refusal) to come to terms with the 'positive' check which inhered in Malthus's defence of Haileybury led to a related (and again, probably intentional) misunderstanding of his agenda. If the point was to force students to understand fully the consequences of falling prey to temptation, it stood to reason that unruly students should be given the fullest opportunity to behave in a manner that warranted expulsion. Such, at least, was Malthus's way of explaining why professors had been content to let previous riots play themselves out, before ridding the school of the ringleaders. To many shareholders, in contrast, such actions were signs of timidity, if not worse. It 'appeared extraordinary' to Lord Elphinstone, for instance, 'that not one of the professors should have ever interfered to quell the disturbances but had stood aside, as if to see to what length they might be carried'.[27]

In the debate over Haileybury in 1817, shareholders often cited polemical passages from Malthus's pamphlet as a means of diverting attention from undisciplined students to insubordinate professors. Randall Jackson accused Malthus of leading 'a knot of schoolmasters and five brother clergymen' who were bent on usurping the directors' constitutional powers, and Joseph Hume similarly criticised 'the insubordinate language to the Directors by Mr. professor Malthus, who was paid by the Company, and ought to have conducted himself with more decorum to his employers'. In 1824, during a further round of debate, another shareholder criticised Haileybury professors on account of their light teaching load ('some had but four hours' labour in the week, others two hours in two days, and the rest of the week open'), and urged them to teach evening classes to help keep students out of trouble.[28]

This torrent of shareholder hostility quickly led Malthus to realise that in order to control the behaviour of his students, it was also necessary to control the behaviour of those parents who were 'irritated at the merited punishment of their sons'. Large sections of *Statements* blamed bad parenting, not bad teaching, on the riots at Haileybury, as when Malthus suggested that many students intentionally misbehaved in order to get out of a career path their parents had forced them to pursue. Such children, he claimed, made their professors pay for the resentment they felt at being sent to India against their will, since they preferred 'expulsion, on occasion of some general disturbance ... to an open and manly rejection of an appointment which is considered by their parents as so valuable'. To support this claim, he reported instances in which students who had been temporarily suspended from the college returned with 'letters containing expressions of ... the most anxious desire to proceed to India', followed by a new round of behaviour that was guaranteed to lead to expulsion.[29] Parents also impeded the college's mission when they lavishly provided their children with gifts, which blurred the contrast between Haileybury's 'elevating' luxuries and those on offer in India. It was with this in mind that Malthus's ally Robert Grant condemned the 'profuse indulgence' and 'profuse sums of money' given to students by their relatives while they were at the college.[30]

Such considerations led Malthus to discern a direct tie between the quality of education at Haileybury and the East India Company's suspect history of patronage-inspired corruption. Many East India shareholders, he lamented, wished for nothing more than to 'get their children off their hands as early as possible, with little regard of the consequences to the Company'. These parents were especially likely to gripe when they found their child delivered back to them, having been deemed by the teaching staff to be 'headstrong' or 'refractory'. Malthus hoped, in such cases, that the 'positive check' of expulsion would force parents to face up to the corrupting consequences of the company's patronage system, just as starvation cruelly taught paupers the lesson of unrestrained sex. These parents would suffer directly as a result of their child's misbehaviour, instead of being blind to the future harm he would cause to the company's constitution and the suffering he would cause to innocent subjects in India. Nor, Malthus was quick to add, was their own suffering really all that terrible. They still received dividends on their stock (this was, after all, their nominal reason for buying it); and as for their unfortunate child, he was confident that '[s]ome employments may be found at home even for a very feeble capacity'.[31]

If these parallels between the 'positive checks' of starving paupers and expelled pupils was clear, the point where this analogy broke down was also painfully obvious: 'nature' weeded out the weakest people in the first case, and politically vulnerable professors did the weeding out in the second. At least as far as the narrow question of expulsion was concerned, however, Malthus was able to fend off repeated attacks from disgruntled shareholders by relying on important allies at the Court of Directors, and by appealing to the need for shareholders and staff to provide a unified front against the threat of outside government regulation. The latter strategy had been enough to neutralise shareholder opposition to the college in 1813, when the company's charter was up for renewal and public scrutiny of its affairs was intense. That year, in fact, Haileybury's staff secured additional autonomy from the directors, in the form of a 'certificate of good conduct' from the college as a prerequisite for service in India and an independent appeals judge (the Bishop of London, a close ally of Malthus) for all expulsions. In 1817, Malthus enjoyed the support of the Evangelical director Robert Grant, who envisioned the college as a training ground for missionaries.[32] That year Grant, who concluded a rousing speech in defence of Malthus by proclaiming the 'grand principle of their empire... to be a love of conferring rather than of receiving benefits', shamed enough shareholders into submission to prevent an inquiry into the college's affairs.[33]

Malthus's very strategy of letting each new crop of students discover for themselves the consequences of delinquency, however, had the side effect of keeping Haileybury's fate perpetually up in the air. Within days of the vote against the inquiry in 1817, the *Times* reported that the college's principal had been 'chased, with very opprobrious language, by a dog with a kettle tied to his tail; one of the Tutors was beaten; [and] the Steward had his head broken'. Although no expulsions resulted in this case, further disturbances in 1822 led to another round of expulsions the following year, which in turn bred further dissension among company shareholders regarding the future of the college. Although Haileybury again survived the test (this time by a vote of 400 to 272), the *Times* concluded with some justice that 'this feeble majority, upon which... so unreasonably vast institution depends, should tend to correct its errors and modify its extravagances'.[34]

The fact that expulsions consistently led shareholders to challenge professorial authority led Malthus to consider measures that might produce more co-operation between parents and professors in the proper training of the Haileybury students. In his *Statements* he wistfully contrasted the recriminations surrounding discipline at Haileybury with the way these things were done at 'the

Universities, and at great schools'. There, when tutors asked parents 'quietly to remove' students who were misbehaving, 'such hints are always taken as commands, and it is no doubt a most effectual mode of... preventing the spread of mischief, without exciting public sensation'. In the short term, Malthus saw little hope of experiencing such well-mannered parent-teacher interactions at Haileybury, for the simple reason that few parents would put up with the loss of their child's dearly-purchased Indian appointment without a fight.[35] In the longer term, however, his implicit comparison of Haileybury with Oxbridge and the 'great schools' suggested a possible method of getting shareholders voluntarily to put the greater interests of Indian government above their immediate selfish desires. This method pointed to an aggressive marketing campaign to convince parents that Haileybury, far from being an annoying obstacle to plunder, had the power of enriching the lives and the future careers of their children. Once they valued the college as a worthwhile investment in its own right, they would be willing to factor its short-term drawbacks into the price of entry.

To bring this point home to shareholders, Malthus practised in his *Statements* the same consumerism he was starting to preach in his *Essay on Population*. Using language that would not be out of place in a modern college brochure, he went out of his way to emphasise the many unique advantages that Haileybury offered to students who were about to set off for India. Its high admission standards meant that new students would not have to mix with lower-class children; its tuition of £100 was a bargain in comparison to other public schools; and its reputation for disciplinary problems was an unwarranted slander based on a few 'temporary ebullitions'. Malthus concluded, with the sweeping assurance of a seasoned public-relations professional, that

> a considerable proportion of the students of the East-India college, who have proceeded to India, have left it with more improved understandings, a greater quantity of useful knowledge, fitted for the early discharge of public business, and more steady habits of good conduct, than could be found among any set of young men, taken... at the same age, from any place of public education in Europe.[36]

All this added up to an impassioned, if only partially successful, effort to present Haileybury as a status symbol that was valuable enough in itself to deserve the support of parents despite the fact that not all of its graduates made it to their destined positions in India. And such risks, as Robert Grant reminded shareholders in 1817, should apply just as readily to the human capital of children as to shares in any other commercial undertaking: 'what was the mighty risk and danger of sending a lad to Hertford, which was not infinitely overbalanced by advantages?'[37]

Formalising moral restraint: examination problems

Despite his temporary success at protecting Haileybury from its enemies, Malthus was not completely content with the college's existing methods of turning boys into men. He further suggested in *Statements* that an improved system of competitive exams would amplify the educational potential of moral restraint by adding a further 'distinction' to the college's arsenal (for those who survived the test), and by introducing a further 'positive check' (by weeding out those who did not). Exams had been an important part of the college's program since 1813, when for the first time a student's academic performance and not the 'Rank' of his patron determined his appointment in India. Malthus praised this system as enabling professors to 'mark with sufficient precision the industrious and the indolent, the able and the deficient, the well-disposed and the turbulent'. But he encouraged the company to raise the stakes of the exam, and further fray the connection between patrons and jobs, by stocking the college with more students than there were appointments, then using the exam to weed out the worst of these students. 'If the Directors were to appoint one-fifth every year, beyond the number finally to go out', he argued, this would make an appointment 'a prize to be contended for, not a property already possessed' – hence, as it were, 'overpopulating' the crop of students to insure a stronger class of survivors.[38]

Although the logic of this scheme was wholly consistent with Malthus's defence of combining 'distinction' and expulsion to get the most out of his students, its institutional ramifications betrayed sharp tensions within his wider goal of moral restraint. By trying to shift the grounds for expulsion from the category of disciplinary outrage to that of academic incompetence, Malthus found himself moving from one horn to the other of a dilemma which Mary Poovey, following Foucault, has identified as 'the paradox of disciplinary individualism'. In Poovey's construction, early Victorians tried to solve this paradox (which she defines as an effort to 'instil a *collective* sense of *individual* responsibility') in one of two ways. The first, favoured by the Malthusian evangelical minister Thomas Chalmers, was to rely on charisma to subordinate the personal responsibility of others to the greater good; the second, favoured by the Malthusian sanitary reformer Edwin Chadwick, was to accomplish this feat using the coercive powers of bureaucracy. But neither attempt, she concludes, was successful on its own terms. Chalmers's charisma soon became institutionalised in a manner that made it hard to distinguish his charity efforts from the New Poor Law, and Chadwick's hardy faith in rational bureaucracy soon yielded a system that relied far more on personal persuasion than on formal rules.[39]

The fact that both protagonists in Poovey's story were Malthusians is not coincidental, since Malthus himself spent an entire career shuttling between their two different responses to the paradox of 'disciplinary individualism'. At Haileybury, his central defence of expulsion as a means of amplifying the consequences of delinquency reflected a 'charismatic' response: foreknowledge of possible removal would enhance students' respect for the personal authority of their professors. His additional proposal to weed out one-fifth of each incoming class, in contrast, reflected a bureaucratic response, relying on numerical grades and the 'strict impartiality' of the graders.[40] Although Malthus was able to keep these two different motivating strategies in his head (or at least in his book) simultaneously, such was not the case with others who took an interest in Haileybury's fate. They either assumed that Malthus's advocacy of a more bureaucratic college was in reality a ploy to add to the professors' personal authority; or they assumed that his bureaucratic vision could never succeed unless it was supported by the coercive powers of the British government – in which case Haileybury itself would no longer be needed.

Between 1817 and 1853, the fate of competitive exams as a solution to Indian patronage depended on the ability of this latter perspective to win a political following. Such a following was notably absent in the initial response to Malthus's proposed 'weeding out' scheme, which was uniformly hostile even among Haileybury's supporters. In 1817 it was difficult for people to imagine an institutional setting, at least in England and certainly in a chartered company, in which bureaucratic authority could be anything other than a thinly-veiled grab at patronage. Jacob Bosanquet, who otherwise defended Malthus, suspected that his 'plan of adding six more students for the purpose of plucking an equal number, in order to excite competition' was an attempt 'to transfer the civil patronage of the company to the professors of the college'.[41] He did not need to remind shareholders of the obvious similarities between this alleged attempt and the alleged effort by Fox and Burke in 1783, again in the name of efficiency and impartiality, to transfer Indian power from the company to the state.

Concerns about patronage, and the personal authority that came with it, again overrode any possible benefits from a more bureaucratic educational system when the company's charter was up for renewal in 1833. That year Thomas Macaulay and Charles Wynn proposed, as a rider to the charter, an entrance exam at Haileybury which would weed out three-fourths of the applicants for admission, without interfering with the directors' privilege of selecting the applicant pool. The proposal increased the 'overpopulation' of nominated candidates from 20% to 400%, but retained the same principle Malthus had proposed in 1817; and Haileybury itself was to remain as a further weeding-out facility for those candidates who had passed the entrance.[42] Although this proposal formally passed both Houses as part of the final India Bill, it was never established in practice. Like Malthus, Macaulay found himself in the unfortunate position of trying to persuade directors and shareholders to sacrifice whatever personal gains the patronage system might bring their way, with the only compensation being his promise that the new system would produce 'young men either superior in talents or in diligence to the mass'.[43]

By 1853, when Charles Wood and Charles Trevelyan re-opened the question of company patronage, its shareholders were more vulnerable to being nudged towards forsaking their personal authority than they had been in past debates; if Macaulay's proposed reforms had been at the cutting edge of political opinion twenty years earlier, Wood could now present his reform as a moderate alternative to calls for abolishing the company altogether. What had moved Wood's reforms to the centre of political opinion was a growing acceptance by Whig politicians of the principle of competitive examination as a path to civil service reform.[44] In the short term, this development prevented the company's traditional appeals against competitive exams from generating much political support. In the longer term, it paved the way for a transfer of power from the company to the state, which would be accomplished in 1858. What had begun as a gentle nudge in 1853 became less gentle when Wood and Trevelyan turned from simply restraining the abuse of patronage to abolishing patronage as a system of selecting candidates for the civil service.

When Wood first looked into Indian civil service reform in 1852, he assumed it would be possible to abolish patronage simply by taking Macaulay's prior proposal to its logical extreme. Instead of calling for the directors to select a surplus of candidates for admission, which would have diluted the effects of their patronage without formally taking it away, he proposed to open competitive exams for admission to

Haileybury to all who cared to apply. All prospective company servants, regardless of family connections, would be equal in the eyes of their examiners. One noteworthy outcome of this scheme was that the Haileybury professors, as administrators of the entrance tests, would have replaced their directors in the act of dispensing patronage – hence confirming the directors' earlier fears about Malthus's ulterior reason for promoting competitive exams. This transfer of power from the directors to the college was fully consistent with Trevelyan's reform philosophy, which was to retain the moral influence of patronage but move it outside the Cabinet (or in this case the company's executive branch). Tutors at the East India College, who were hired for life by the directors, occupied a place in the company that was identical to the position to be filled by Cabinet-appointed Civil Service Commissioners; the only difference was that the Haileybury staff would provide the added bonus of what Trevelyan called in 1853 'a very satisfactory system of special instruction for the Indian Civil Service'.[45]

Within weeks of defending Haileybury in those terms, however, Trevelyan was won over to a new method of applying the principle of competitive examination to the India Civil Service that eventually eliminated any need for Haileybury. With prodding from educational reformers at Harrow and Oxford, Trevelyan decided that the breadth of a liberal Oxbridge education was to be preferred over the narrower training at the East India College as a criterion for choosing civil servants. He consequently convinced Wood to include a clause in the 1853 India Bill allowing the President of the Board of Control to determine the matter of civil service reform at a later date, in order to see how more University men might be recruited to serve in India. In the gradual evolution of the new scheme, the maximum age for taking the entrance exam was first raised to 23, which allowed Oxbridge graduates to compete with the usual crop of teenagers for an extra two years of special Indian training.[46] From there, it was only a matter of time before Wood closed the college for being 'altogether unsuited to the instruction of gentlemen, many of whom may have passed through the full course of education at one or the other of the universities', and what had been an entrance exam to Haileybury turned into a final hurdle for University graduates to pass before heading directly to India.[47]

Conclusion

On the face of it, the closure of Haileybury in 1854 defeated everything Malthus had fought for in *Statements Regarding the East-India College*, which was nothing if not a plea for the college's survival. It could be argued, however, that handing the selection of Indian servants over to a state-appointed Civil Service Commission actually brought to full fruition Malthus's original aim to employ moral restraint as an educational philosophy. This suggestion gains in plausibility when it is recalled that one of the striking features of the civil service reforms was the extent to which they internalised the system of rewards and criteria of selection that were in use at Cambridge and Oxford. In this sense, Wood's reform simply replaced Haileybury's unco-operative patrons, who had refused to accept the rules of the college as a necessary expense, with a new set of patrons who were happy to play the game of college admissions as they had been defined by the Universities and elite public schools. The moral restraint of Indian patronage did not disappear in 1853, it simply resurfaced in a stronger form in Oxbridge. The same conclusion applies, in the realm of population theory, to the New Poor Law, which was only superficially a far cry from Malthus's call for the poor laws to be abolished in order to make way for the lessons of 'nature'. At least in theory, the commissioners under the new poor law were simply creating artificial circumstances in which the 'natural' laws of political economy would operate more efficiently.[48]

This evaluation rescues Malthus's appeal to moral restraint in a narrow sense, but does not address the more general problem with his assumption that a free market could 'naturally' secure restrained behaviour without constant and arbitrary assistance from the state. Especially in the context of Empire, in which the threat constantly resurfaced of servants on the scene subverting the more 'restrained' decrees passed down from London, the hope of permanently preventing recourse to arbitrary restraint was never realised. Burke's vision of waves of youthful British servants sowing their seeds in Indian soil was an exaggeration even when it was written, and increasingly lost relevance as an accurate depiction of Indian government as the nineteenth century progressed. But as a metaphor for the institutional problem of restraining imperial desire, the Burkean trope of sublime excess is at least as evocative as the Malthusian theme of uncoerced restraint.

Notes

1   See, for example, Boyd Hilton, *The Age of Atonement: The Influence of Evangelicalism on Social and Economic Thought, 1795-1865* (Oxford: Oxford University Press, 1988); Linda Colley, *Britons: Forging the Nation 1707-1837* (New Haven: Yale University Press, 1992).

2. See especially Catherine Gallagher, 'The Body Versus the Social

Body in the Works of Thomas Malthus and Henry Mayhew',
Representations xiv (1986), 83–106.

3. See Geoffrey Gilbert, 'Economic Growth and the Poor in Malthus'
Essay on Population', *History of Political Economy* xii (1980), 84–96.

4. Smith, *An Inquiry into the Nature and Causes of the Wealth of Nations*
(1776; Oxford: Oxford University Press, 1976), 619. See Timothy L.
Alborn, *Conceiving Companies: Joint-Stock Politics in Victorian
England* (London: Routledge, 1998), 24–7.

5. *Ibid.*, 637, 640. The £1400 share price referred to the going
premium on a £1000 share in the Company as of 1776; after 1773
this was the minimum holding necessary to be able to vote for
directors.

6. Burke, *Speeches* (Boston: Little, Brown and Co., 1865), II, 462–3.
See Sara Suleri, *The Rhetoric of English India* (Chicago: University of
Chicago Press, 1992), chapter 2.

7. Peter Marshall, *Problems of Empire: Britain and India 1757-1813*
(London: George Allen and Unwin, 1968), 33–42.

8. This section of the chapter expands on arguments I make in *op. cit.*
(ref. 4), 31–5.

9. Other measures put in place by Wellesley and William Bentinck, and
accepted without a fight by the Court of Directors, included
enforcing a regular schedule of promotion in the service and
requiring revenue officers to submit accounts to the Board.

10. For background on Haileybury, especially during the period
1811–1817, see Patricia James, *Population Malthus, His Life and
Times* (London: Routledge and Kegan Paul, 1979), 214–22, 228–43;
and Keith Tribe, 'Professors Malthus and Jones: Political Economy at
the East India College 1806-1858', *European Journal of the History of
Economic Thought* ii (1995), 327–38.

11. *Times*, 28 November 1811; 20 December 1811.

12. James, *op. cit.* (ref. 10), 214, 230–3.

13. Cited in *ibid.*, 231.

14. Malthus, *Statements respecting the East-India College* (London, 1817)
in *The Pamphlets of Thomas Robert Malthus* (New York: Kelley,
1970), 241-6. This was in effect a second edition of his much less
widely-circulated *Letter to Lord Grenville*, published in 1813.

15. Malthus, *An Essay on the Principle of Population* (1803; Cambridge:
Cambridge University Press, 1992), 9.

16. *Ibid.*, 213. Donald Winch identifies this passage as evidence of
Malthus's 'Paleyite utilitarianism': Winch, *Riches and Poverty: An
Intellectual History of Political Economy in Britain, 1750-1834*
(Cambridge: Cambridge University Press, 1996), 243–4.

17. Cited in Gilbert, *op. cit.* (ref. 3), 92, 94. Malthus had hoped to publish this edition of the *Essay* in 1815, but he was delayed by the disturbances at Haileybury: see James, *op. cit.* (ref. 10), 233.

18. Winch discusses Malthus's views on working-class education in his introduction to Malthus, *op. cit.* (ref. 15), xvii–xviii.

19. Malthus, *op. cit.* (ref. 14), 255, 279.

20. *Ibid.*, 307–8.

21. For a discussion of Smith's influence (including *Theory of Moral Sentiments*) on Malthus, see Winch, *op. cit.* (ref. 16), 237–40.

22. Malthus, *op. cit.* (ref. 14), 273–4.

23. Malthus, *op. cit.* (ref. 15), 190. For a feminist reading which relates Malthus's views on 'savage' colonies to his moral theories see Randi Davenport, 'Thomas Malthus and Maternal Bodies Politic: Gender, Race, and Empire', *Women's History Review* iv (1995), 421–5.

24. Malthus, *op. cit.* (ref. 14), 262, 267, 317.

25. *Ibid.*, 279, 298–9, 307.

26. *Times*, 7 January 1817, 21 February 1817.

27. *Times*, 5 March 1817.

28. *Times*, 7 February 1817, 26 February 1817, 28 February 1824.

29. Malthus, *op. cit.* (ref. 14), 303, 288.

30. *Times*, 7 February 1817, 5 March 1817.

31. Malthus, *op. cit.* (ref. 14), 264–5.

32. James, *op. cit.* (ref. 10), 216–7, 221.

33. *Times*, 21 February, 1817.

34. *Times*, 5 March 1817; 9 March 1817; 29 March 1823; 1 April 1824.

35. Malthus, *op. cit.* (ref. 14), 289.

36. *Ibid.*, 271, 260, 274–5.

37. *Times*, 21 February 1817. Robert Grant had earlier observed that only seventeen of 427 students had actually been expelled since Haileybury's establishment, and that five of these had been re-admitted: *Times*, 7 February 1817.

38. Malthus, *op. cit.* (ref. 14), 256, 318n; James, *op. cit.* (ref. 10), 221.

39. Mary Poovey, *Making a Social Body: British Cultural Formation, 1830-1864* (Chicago: Chicago University Press, 1995), ch. 5; 103q.

40. Malthus, *op. cit.* (ref. 14), 273.

41. *Times*, 5 March 1817.

42. C.H. Philips, *The East India Company 1784-1834* (Manchester: Manchester University Press, 1940), 295-6. Philips points out that Wynn's proposal had the potential of sneaking ministerial patronage in through the back door, since it stipulated that if the Directors did not come up with the estimated 160 nominees per year called for by the plan, selection of nominees would revert to the Board of Control.

43. T.B. Macaulay, *Works* (London: Longmans, Green and Co., 1875), VIII, 132; Philips, *op. cit.* (ref. 42), 296–7.

44. As Clive Dewey has observed, 'Sacrifice of the East India company's patronage... appealed to two great Whig traditions: their antipathy, developed over decades of opposition, to executives strong through the exercise of patronage; and their more recently acquired flair for intelligent minimal concession to mass political discontent'. See C.J. Dewey, 'The Education of a Ruling Caste: The Indian Civil Service in the Era of Competitive Examinations', *English Historical Review* lxxxviii (1973), 266.

45. R.J. Moore, 'The Abolition of Patronage in the Indian Civil Service and the Closure of Haileybury College', *Historical Journal* vii (1964), 249.

46. This was substantially the same system that had been proposed by Lord Grenville in 1813, and that had led Malthus to write the first version of his *Statements*. The Company shareholder Douglas Kinnaird had also proposed an open competitive exam in 1823: see *Times*, 18 December 1823.

47. Moore, *op. cit.* (ref. 45), 250–7.

48. See, e.g., Anthony Brundage, *The Making of the New Poor Law: The Politics of Inquiry, Enactment, and Implementation* (New Brunswick, NJ: Rutgers University Press, 1978).

3

The Malthusian Moment

Roy Porter

It is mere alphabetical accident, I suppose, that the names of so many of the great intellectual irritants – those 'realists' who dispense bitter pills to mankind – begin with 'm'. First Moses and Mohammed; then More and Machiavelli, who taught that might was right; then Mandeville for whom private vices were public benefits; and so all the way to Marx, Mao and Marcuse, taking in Malthus *en route*.

Casting his deep shadow over the century of enlightenment, the Revd Thomas Robert Malthus – never *Thomas*, always *Robert*, or *Bob* to his friends – came to the dismal conclusion that the perils of overpopulation were bound to stymie prospects of 'any very great future improvement of society'.[1] Betterment, explained his *An Essay on the Principle of Population* (1798), encouraged breeding, reproduction would then inexorably outstrip food production, and surplus mouths meant misery. 'The work begun by Malthus and completed by Ricardo', judged John Maynard Keynes, 'provide[d] an immensely powerful intellectual foundation to justify the *status quo* ... and to keep us all in order' – or, in Southey's blunt verdict, 'his book [became] the political bible of the rich, the selfish, and the sensual'.[2]

Malthusianism's special attractiveness to reactionaries in an age assuming a Gradgrindian reverence for scientific facts and figures derived from its appeal to iron laws of nature expressed in numbers. Food supplies crept up arithmetically: 2, 4, 6, etc.; human population leapt geometrically: 2, 4, 8, 16, etc. The implication of this simple arithmetic was, as Mr Micawber would have spotted, disaster – that is, the positive checks of famine, war and pestilence. Unless, as later editions stressed, people wised up and pre-empted Nature by employing the salutary preventive check of moral restraint: abstinence and delayed marriage, or misery mitigated. The Malthusian trap was a clever card to play. No-one, the clergyman unfailingly claimed, could be a truer friend of humanity, none more liberal, candid or eager for improvement; it was hardly his fault if

Nature's niggardliness frustrated these goals.[3] There was no arguing with numbers, asserted the man Thomas Love Peacock satirized in his novel *Melincourt* as 'Mr Fax'.[4]

Naturally, this invocation of science's objective decrees was politically motivated, and Malthus's own ideological purposes, while decked out in statistics, were at least explicit in the first edition, which took up the challenge of the French Revolution. All was change:

> The great and unlooked for discoveries that have taken place of late years in natural philosophy; the increasing diffusion of general knowledge from the extension of the art of printing; the ardent and unshackled spirit of inquiry that prevails throughout the lettered, and even unlettered world; the new and extraordinary lights that have been thrown on political subjects, which dazzle, and astonish the understanding; and particularly that tremendous phenomenon in the political horizon the French revolution, which, like a blazing comet, seems destined either to inspire with fresh life and vigour, or to scorch up and destroy the shrinking inhabitants of the earth, have all concurred to lead many able men into the opinion, that we were touching on a period big with the most important changes, changes that would in some measure be decisive of the future fate of mankind.[5]

The champagne fizz of 1789 had inspired intoxicating visions. Revolutionaries dreamt of a heaven on earth, nor did Malthus ever deny the allure of this 'new dawn'.[6] Yet his tone was one not of optimism but admonition: all prophecies of boundless progress were self-defeating.

Enlightenment mercantilist thinking and Paleyan natural theology alike applauded populousness as the pulse of a healthy nation. But, countered Malthus, the laws governing population had never been strictly analysed – least of all by eupeptic prophets of perfectibility like William Godwin, author of the *Enquiry into Political Justice* (1793), and the Marquis de Condorcet, whose *Esquisse d'un Tableau Historique des Progrès de l'Esprit Humain* appeared posthumously in 1795.[7] 'The cause of this neglect on the part of the advocates for the perfectibility of mankind, is not easily accounted for', taunted Malthus, icily scathing about the visionaries' refusal to face facts. 'I have certainly no right to say that they purposely shut their eyes to such arguments.... Yet ... we are all of us too prone to err'.[8]

To dispel such romantic reveries, Malthus presented himself as the champion of realism, faithful to facts and scornful of 'mere conjectures'.[9] He and he alone was training the searchlight of science onto those mechanisms of production and reproduction 'explained in part by Hume, and more at large by Dr Adam Smith'.[10] And what was the verdict when great expectations were thus subjected to demographic actualities? 'Were the rising generation free from the "killing frost" of misery', he observed, 'population must rapidly increase', for affluence would permit earlier marriage and thus lead to bigger families: 'Were every man sure of a comfortable provision for a family, almost every man would have one'.[11] Condorcet had actually taken note of this fact and its potential dangers and, continued Malthus,

> after having described further improvements, he says, "But in this progress of industry and happiness, each generation will be called to more extended enjoyments, and in consequence, by the physical constitution of the human frame, to an increase in the number of individuals. Must not there arrive a period then, when these laws, equally necessary, shall counteract each other?... Will it not mark the limit when all further amelioration will become impossible?"[12]

But having thus glimpsed the monster of overpopulation, Condorcet had looked away. Malthus honoured the *philosophe* for acknowledging that rising numbers were a dilemma not, as traditionally represented, a desideratum, but blamed him for then ducking the big issue. Godwin, for his part, had been even more head in the clouds:

> The system of equality which Mr Godwin proposes, is, without doubt, by far the most beautiful and engaging of any that has yet appeared.... But, alas! that moment can never arrive. The whole is little better than a dream, a beautiful phantom of the imagination.[13]

Godwin and other utopians blamed misery on the *ancien régime*, abolish that, and, hey-presto, what would not be possible? But 'the great error under which Mr Godwin labours throughout his whole work is, the attributing almost all the vices and misery that are seen in civil society to human institutions'.[14] In truth, the real spanner in the works was not government but Nature, and its productive and reproductive economy. 'I think', Malthus proposed, 'I may fairly make two postulata':

> First, That food is necessary to the existence of man.

> Secondly, That the passion between the sexes is necessary, and will remain nearly in its present state.

These two laws ever since we have had any knowledge of mankind, appear to have been fixed laws of our nature.[15]

Increasing geometrically, population inescapably tended to outrun resources and thereby precipitate such crises as famine, epidemics and war. Godwin refused to admit that here lay any real difficulty – 'myriads of centuries of still increasing population may pass away', he was sure, without overpopulation becoming a problem: moreover his favourite solution – 'that the passion between the sexes may in time be extinguished', for people 'will no longer have any motive ... to induce them' – seemed to Malthus frivolous and chimerical.[16] In short, the imbalance of production and reproduction presented an obstacle 'insurmountable in the way to the perfectibility of society', and biology thwarted schemes of universal plenty and social equality: 'I see no way by which man can escape from the weight of this law which pervades all animated nature'.[17]

The *Essay* presaged a dismal future, with Nature ever poised to punish hubris. More constructively if hardly less punitively, subsequent editions suggested that catastrophe could be avoided through what Malthus dubbed 'moral restraint'.[18] Those unable to support families should abstain from marriage or, within marriage, desist from irresponsible gratification. (Malthus of course disapproved of contraception, which was a direct incitement to vice). Reinforcing his earlier call for the abolition of the Poor Law, which he judged self-defeating, the second edition of 1803 conjured up the notorious image of 'Nature's feast' where there was 'no vacant cover' for the poor, who, being uninvited guests, had 'no claim of *right* to the smallest portion of food' – Southey glossed this as a directive to the rich to 'harden their hearts and let the poor starve'.[19]

My task is not to trace the Malthusian controversy in the domains of demographics, political economy, and the natural and human sciences at large – such fields are covered by other essays in this volume. Rather I shall examine how British medical men responded to the *Essay* in the years immediately after its first publication. I take my inspiration from a pioneering article published by William Coleman back in 1980 on the French public health doctor, François Mélier, entitled 'Medicine Against Malthus'.[20]

Mixed reactions might be anticipated.[21] There was much in the *Essay* to which doctors were likely to be sympathetic. Malthus's family itself had a medical tradition – one of his forebears had even been apothecary to the great Thomas Sydenham. Like progressive physicians, Malthus – himself ninth wrangler in 1788 and later a founder-member of the statistical section of the BAAS – valued the numerical approach of William Petty and later political arithmeticians.[22] And he drew extensively upon epidemiological pioneers such as Dr Thomas Short, whose mid-eighteenth century work highlighted the winnowing action of plagues and pestilence.[23] In particular, Malthus himself, though an Anglican cleric – hence Cobbett's immortal gibe 'Parson!'[24] – proposed an astonishingly reductionist model of the human animal. His doctrines, he declared, were based not on the theology of original sin but on the laws of organic life. According to his friend Mrs Schimmelpenninck, the polymath physician Erasmus Darwin styled man 'an eating animal, a drinking animal and a sleeping animal' – presumably amongst his male cronies Darwin substituted a more earthly epithet for 'sleeping'.[25] So blunt a dictum comes hardly unexpectedly from the mouth of a liberal Enlightenment Deist who was a leading light of the Lunar Society.[26] What is *prima facie* more surprising is that Parson Malthus should have embraced no less corporeal a model. William Hazlitt was spot on, as ever, when he observed that 'Mr. Malthus's whole book rests on a malicious supposition, that all mankind (I hope the reader will pardon the grossness of the expression, the subject is a gross one) are like so many animals *in season*'.[27]

Yet Malthus's materialism about the human animal is not so odd after all. Malthus's father, Daniel, was, just like Darwin, a torchbearer of Enlightenment – indeed he personally befriended Rousseau and in true progressive mode had had his son educated by some of the most advanced teachers in the country, including Gilbert Wakefield of the Warrington Academy and William Frend, who tutored him from 1784 at Jesus College, Cambridge (Frend was later expelled for his Jacobinism). Schooled in Lockean philosophy and Hartley's physicalist psychology, young Bob had been groomed by his father to become a philosophical radical – before what might be deemed his oedipal revolt into reaction. The point here is that the *Essay on Population*'s model of man as a consuming and reproducing animal, indeed its quasi-materialistic vision of mind emergent out of matter thanks to the sanctions of struggle, would surely have been, in principle, intellectually congenial to doctors steeped in medical materialism.[28]

Not least, medical writers had already, of course, been confronting the problems Malthus addressed. Thus, seeking to demonstrate that Poor Law outdoor relief aggravated the very problems they were supposed to cure, Joseph Townsend had anticipated Malthus in his *A Dissertation on the Poor Laws*, published in 1786, and in *A Journey Through Spain in the Years 1786 and 1787*, published five years later in 1791. Both works showed that well-meaning attempts to improve society foundered because of man's inordinate procreative instincts. The only recourse, thought Townsend, was to 'leave one appetite to regulate another' and stomach the harsh consequences. Though vicar of Pewsey in Wiltshire, Townsend was probably best known for his extensive medical writings, including *A Guide to Health* (1795) and the popular *The Physicians' Vade Mecum* (1805).[29]

And, of course, as stressed by Maureen McNeil, Erasmus Darwin himself had offered a view of the economy of animated life driven by Nature's superfecundity, with its consequent law of 'eat or be eaten'. Darwin, however, drew from this theatre of struggle not Malthusian pessimism but prospects of progress, maintaining that, through Nature's sanguinary wars, the fittest would survive and happiness triumph via the evolution of superior species. Practising what they respectively preached, the exuberant Darwin, for his part, exercised no personal moral restraint, siring fourteen children and growing immensely fat, while Malthus on the other hand prudently delayed marriage till he was thirty-eight and produced just three.[30]

Yet medical men would surely also have found much in Malthus that jarred. For one thing, Georgian doctors routinely commended procreative activity for the individual and populousness for the state. For another, Malthus's views implied a therapeutic fatalism in the face of the positive check of disease which was bound to have affronted medical *amour propre*. Like the poor, plagues and pestilences were always with us as part of Providence's dispensation, even, Malthus seemed to be saying, a perhaps kindlier means of culling than starvation. Rumour had it, indeed, that Malthus was thus opposed to smallpox vaccination.[31] Doctors could not easily endorse a doctrine which viewed disease as inescapable and even salutary.

Moreover the self-image of vocal cadres within the medical profession – especially those Scottish-educated Dissenters debarred from the Royal College oligarchies – was politically liberal and progressive.[32] Just as clinical expertise would treat individual patients, so the profession should serve as doctors to society, forming a technocratic vanguard. Not for practitioners the parson's gloomy notions of Providence and theological justifications of the ways of God to man.

All that, however, is conjecture – it is time to get down to Malthusian brass tacks and inquire as to the actual responses of doctors. Did they make a distinctive contribution to the Malthusian debate?

The first doctor to go into print was the rather obscure Charles Hall, born perhaps in 1745 and dying around 1825.[33] It seems he studied in Leiden in the 1760s and he possibly published in 1785 *The Medical Family Instructor*, a typical home-help book of its day. Early in the nineteenth century, Hall was ruined by a law suit, ending up in the Fleet. Though his friends offered to pay for his release, he deemed that he had been unjustly treated, and so resolved to die in prison.

In 1805 he brought out *The Effects of Civilization on the People in European States*, later adding to it an Appendix entitled: *Observations on the Principal Conclusion in Mr. Malthus's Essay on Population.*[34] Like Malthus, Hall was haunted by the spectre of poverty; the doctor, however, insisted that the root of the problem lay in the villainous political system. Society had become divided into two nations, rich and poor. The latter lived in wretchedness and suffered a much higher death rate. Exact calculation was impossible, Hall admitted, but 'it seems probable that the deaths of the poor are to those of the rich as two to one, in proportion to the numbers of each'. The occupations of the poor were deleterious to their health; their moral education was neglected; their minds were uncultivated; their sports were reviled, their lot was insupportable. All this he laid at the door of an unjust and exploitative system of civilization.[35]

Grain shortages such as those peaking in the 1790s were not to be blamed on Nature but were the consequence of politico-economic mismanagement. Too many workers were quitting the land for manufactures and the towns, leading to scarcity. Dearth would cease and plenty return if the poor were granted access to the soil. Agrarian redistribution would reduce dependency on a cash economy, ever subject to market fluctuations:

> It is an essential liberty that a man enjoy the fruits of his own labour, but in fact eight-tenths of the people consume only one-eighth of the produce. The mechanism of this deprivation is money.

> The poor cannot eat without money. They cannot get money without labour. Those, therefore, that are in possession of money, or the necessaries of life, have the command of the labour of the poor, by having the power of withholding the necessaries of life from them.[36]

Civilization – that is, emergent industrial capitalism – thus

encouraged and sustained a pernicious inequality which was hurtful
to health:

> The sum, therefore, of the effects of civilization, in most civilized
> states, is to enable a few of mankind to attain all possible enjoyments
> both of mind and body, that their nature is susceptible of; but at the
> expense, and by depriving the bulk of mankind of the necessaries
> and comforts of life.[37]

The answer? Cease sacrificing bees to drones, and instead restore
land to the people and labourers to the land. The egalitarianism
which Malthus thought impossible Hall held imperative.[38]

Indeed, in his *Appendix* the doctor turned explicitly to Malthus,
underlining their differences. Respecting poverty, he noted that
Malthus 'does not consider civilization as chargeable with any thing
on this account, because, as he says, the same want and misery must
necessarily happen in every system'. That was false. Politics played its
part. Land redistribution was the answer. Three and a half acres
would support five people. Thus England could sustain 140 millions,
which, allowing for a doubling every 20 years, would give eighty
years' respite. That period could be extended by colonization abroad
and regulation of marriages at home – a measure acceptable in an
egalitarian state in which everybody was affected equally. Admittedly,
as Malthus had pointed out, one day 'the whole world ... will be fully
peopled; ... but this period must be very remote, and ... we ought not
to anticipate the evil by any systems or practices of our own'.[39]
Overall, Hall concluded, in rather Painite terms:

> A part of the people, and especially the smaller part, cannot have a
> right to induce a state of misery and mortality on the great body of
> the nation.... civilization, therefore, is chargeable with anticipating,
> at least, the evils, and bringing them on the people, long before they
> would otherwise have been afflicted with them.[40]

The ruling order first immiserated the poor and then washed its
hands by blaming Nature and (complained Hall) by implication
God. Malthus's verdict that a man who cannot support his family
must be 'doomed to starve' was 'not only inhuman to the last degree,
but unjust and iniquitous', for 'It is not true that he has *doomed
himself,* or that nature has doomed *him and his family to starve;* that
cruel doom is brought on him by the rich.' Hall's book was
torpedoed by the periodical press before sinking almost without
trace, though it must have had some continuing standing in socialist
circles, since it was reprinted in 1850.[41]

My second medical critic is Thomas Jarrold.[42] Born in Manningtree in Essex in 1770 and probably a Dissenter, he was educated at Edinburgh University where he took his M. D., going on to practise in Stockport and later in Manchester where he rubbed along with the manufacturing community. Amongst his writings were *Anthropologia, or Dissertations on the Form and Colour in Man* (1808) and other works on education, character, and the problem of poverty.[43]

In *Dissertations on Man, Philosophical, Physiological and Political; in answer to Mr. Malthus's 'Essay on the Principle of Population*, Jarrold scored many points. Had the clergyman not heard of the Biblical injunction: 'be fruitful and multiply'? The Malthusian ratios were phoney. Under capitalist agriculture, food supply was by no means as inelastic as Malthus supposed. It went without saying that no nation grew more food than it needed. It was all a matter of supply and demand, as with every other commodity. No one expected that a rising population would go *unclothed*, for the woollen and cotton industries would naturally develop to meet rising demand. The same held good for grain. Malthus had set the cart before the horse: 'in place of saying, population increases where subsistence increases, it would be more correct to say, subsistence increases because population increases'.[44]

Malthus had made medical mistakes as well. For instance, Jarrold queried the reality of some of the checks, in particular what Malthus termed 'vice'. In truth, Jarrold argued, donning his public health hat, drunkenness and prostitution had little effect on numbers, nor for that matter did so-called unhealthy trades. An enthusiast for industrialization, Jarrold held (contrary to Hall) that child labour was positively good for infants. The environment found in factories was healthy, largely on account of the hot atmosphere and high concentrations of carbon dioxide.[45]

Above all, Jarrold took Malthus to task on a basic issue. Like Hall, he accused him of wilfully confusing avoidable and unavoidable evils. 'Common diseases and unwholesome seasons are beyond the controul of man', he noted, 'but war is a voluntary act'. Malthus's tactic of attributing all social inequalities to Nature was pure mystification. Jarrold exploded at the notorious passage about the poor having no invitation to Nature's feast: 'at nature's mighty feast, none are bishops, but all are men; there is no distinction; all that are invited are at liberty to partake, and the life of a guest is sacred: to be invited to the same table, implies equality; and to possess life is to possess the invitation'.[46]

Misery was not the *natural* lot of the human race: 'there is no physical cause of war, none of famine, none of pestilence'. Such calamaties stemmed from knavery or folly: 'Pestilence commonly arises out of some act of human folly, or is the consequence of ignorance. War is the parent of pestilence'.[47] Man was thus the agent of his own destruction. Doubtless Malthus was correct to point to the prevalence of misery, but that did not prove its necessity:

> Man has sufficient liberty, sufficient power, to keep down the population of any country to any standard he may please by violence and bloodshed; but God has not appointed him to that task; he is not an executioner by nature; and the office never becomes him.[48]

Quite specifically, Jarrold held that Malthus's prophesy of overpopulation was unfounded. Increase was checked by many forces. Savage tribes were too warlike to expand. In civilized societies, various groups – from prostitutes to professors – produced few offspring: 'thus we find a large part of the community that does not require the operation of vice, misery, or moral restraint, to prevent its increase'.[49]

Fertility was not a biological constant but a social construct, precisely because, so Jarrold insisted, 'man is not a mere animal'. *Pace* Malthus, in matters like sexuality, mankind 'stands apart from brutes'. Reproduction depended upon circumstances, differing from nation to nation, amongst distinct ranks within a single nation, and fluctuating over the course of history. Plague had disappeared from Europe and environmental improvements like fen drainage were reducing the grip of disease.[50]

In an advanced society, a rising population posed no danger, since 'misery has ever been the consequence and the scourge of ignorance and depravity, knowledge its corrective'.[51] And in any case, *pace* Malthus, advances in prosperity and civilization typically brought a *drop* in the birth-rate. A government which enriched its people and tackled misery might even have to take steps against dwindling numbers. Civilized people bred less, for, *pace* Malthus, 'the influence of the mind extends to the propagation of the species'. 'As the faculties of the mind are unemployed, as the man sinks down towards the animal, he is prolific; as he ascends above them, his fruitfulness decreases'.[52]

Thus Hall and Jarrold both attacked Malthus but from diametrically opposite positions. For Hall, hunger and poverty were the progeny of capitalism, not Nature. For Jarrold, the march of modern capitalist society offered an escape from those problems. Hall asserted that political action would eradicate poverty; Jarrold believed the overpoplation threat would wither away with growing prosperity. In either case, Malthus was accused of the fatalism consequent upon naturalizing set-ups which were essentially contingent, historical and political. Against Malthus's degrading vision, Both Hall and Jarrold defended the dignity of man and the designs of God. And both looked forward to better things – on an almost millennial note Jarrold concluded: 'I cannot give up the idea that the period is hastening when the condition of mankind will be far better than it now is .... Already I fancy I have seen the first dawning of this wished-for morning'.[53] There is perhaps an irony in the fact that the clergyman had recourse to ideological arguments from science and medicine, whereas his medical opponents were more inclined to draw upon history and hegemony.

I cannot here trace all the medical responses to Malthus but, so far as I can judge, few if any endorsed his model of the mighty pressures of population. For instance Michael Ryan, author of sundry works on medical jurisprudence, mineral waters, prostitution and obstetrics and also of *The Philosophy of Marriage, in its Social, Moral, and Physical Relations* (1843), ridiculed his theories.[54] Having noted that 'the increase of family without the means of subsistence is a fertile source of anxiety and pauperism', he nevertheless insisted that 'it remains to be proved, whether there is a superabundant population in any civilized country at present; and whether the productions of the animal and vegetable kingdoms are insufficient for the aliment of mankind in general'. After all, the world was six thousand years old and still three-quarters empty.[55]

'This conclusion', Ryan maintained, is totally opposed to the erroneous hypothesis of a benevolent and philanthropic political economist, the late Rev. Mr. Malthus'. Malthus's recommendation of 'celibacy to the age of twenty-eight to thirty years' was not just impractical but a recipe for vice. Luckily it was unnecessary too, since there was no evidence supporting Malthus's pressure of population. Ryan deplored the fact 'the Westminster political economists' – he named 'Bentham, Ricardo, Place, Mill, Tooke, Brougham, Miss Martineau, and others of minor note' – had become 'zealous disciples of Malthus'. This had led to 'grossly immoral men', on pretext of solving Malthus's dilemma, to go round distributing 'the most infamous handbills throughout the large manufacturing districts in England, which purported to contain "the important information for the working classes, how to regulate the number of a family"'. Thus Malthus had actually triggered the increase of vice.[56]

•

May I offer three conclusions to this simple sketch? First, we need to know far more about medical discourses on sex and reproduction in the era before Malthus. Malthus's roots in economics and demographics have been laid bare; but how far did his models of human biology and the sanctions of disease emerge from earlier *medical* thinking?

Second, it is interesting that, so far as I know, Malthus had no conspicuous and vocal early medical supporters. What does this tell us about the politics of early nineteenth-century medicine?

Third, it is noteworthy that medical refutations of Malthus were so bent on exposing his false naturalizing strategy. For both Hall and Jarrold, mankind's past, present and prospects were to be understood not in terms of a reductionist biomedical model but as products of culture and history.

I close on a sad tailnote. In 1804, in a letter to his student son in Edinburgh, the distinguished Liverpool physician Dr James Currie related the story of a lunatic whose reason gave way after indulging in speculations on the perfectibility of man. Currie, who had publicly praised Malthus's *Essay*, felt that it was incumbent upon him to explain to his poor patient the principle of population. The lunatic's reaction? He next produced 'a scheme for enlarging the surface of the globe, and a project for an act of parliament for this purpose, in a letter addressed to Mr. Pitt'. To prove *this* would not solve the problem, Currie then gave the poor fellow Malthus's quarto. The result was all too predictable. He read it twice – the second time out loud – and then, after a few anguished days, lay down and died. 'At the moment that I write this', Currie concluded, 'his copy of Malthus is in my sight; and I cannot look at it but with extreme emotion'. This seems like the ultimate positive check.[57]

Notes

1. Thomas Robert Malthus, *An Essay on the Principle of Population as it Affects the Future Improvement of Society, With Remarks on the Speculations of Mr Godwin, M. Condorcet, And Other Writers* (London: J. Johnson, 1798), Preface, iii. I cite the facsimile reprint: London: Macmillan, 1966.
   For a definitive biography, see Patricia James, *Population Malthus: His Life and Times* (London: Routledge & Kegan Paul, 1979), 1f. I wish to thank Michèle Stokes for her invaluable assistance in researching this article.
2. For Keynes, see Kenneth Smith, *The Malthusian Controversy* (London: Routledge and Paul, 1951), 37; Robert Southey, review of Malthus in *Annual Review* (January, 1804), reprinted in Andrew Pyle (ed.), *Population: Contemporary Responses to Thomas Malthus* (Bristol: Thoemmes Press, 1994), 129. See also Harold A. Boner, *Hungry Generations. The Nineteenth-Century Case Against Malthusianism* (New York: King's Crown Press, Columbia University, 1955), 50.
3. For expositions of Malthus's basic ideas, see J. R. Bonar, *Malthus and his Work* (reprint: London: Frank Cass, 1966); Donald Winch, *Malthus* (Oxford and New York: Oxford University Press, 1987).
4. *The Novels of Thomas Love Peacock*, edited with introductions and notes by David Garnett (London: Rupert Hart-Davis, 1948), 103f.
5. Malthus, *An Essay*, 1–2.
6. William Wordsworth, *The Prelude*, xi, lines 108–9 in J. Wordsworth, M. H. Abrams and S. Gill (eds), *William Wordsworth, the Prelude 1799, 1805, 1850* (London: W. W. Norton and Co., 1979), 397 (1805 version).
7. For such radicals, see Marilyn Butler, *Romantics, Rebels and Reactionaries: English Literature and its Background 1760-1830* (Oxford and New York: Oxford University Press, 1981); Frank E. Manuel and Fritzie P. Manuel, *Utopian Thought in a Western World* (Cambridge, Mass.: Belknap Press, 1979); Clive Emsley, *British Society and the French Wars 1793-1815* (London: Macmillan, 1979).
8. Malthus, *An Essay*, 8–9.
9. Malthus, *An Essay*, 10.
10. Malthus, *An Essay*, 8.
11. Malthus, *An Essay*, 151.
12. Malthus, *An Essay*, 152.
13. Malthus, *An Essay*, 174–5.
14. Malthus, *An Essay*, 176.

15. Malthus, *An Essay*, 11–12.
16. William Godwin, *An Enquiry Concerning Political Justice and its Influence on General Virtue and Happiness* (London: G. G. J. and J. Robinson, 1793). For Godwin, see Don Locke, *A Fantasy of Reason: The Life and Thought of William Godwin* (London and Boston: Routledge and Kegan Paul, 1980).
17. Malthus, *An Essay*, 16–17.
18. For discussion of moral restraint, see Winch, *Malthus*, 38.
19. Thomas Robert Malthus, *An Essay on the Principle of Population: A View of Its Past and Present Effects on Human Happiness, with an Inquiry into our prospects respecting the Future Removal of the Evils which it Occasions*, 2nd edn (London: J. Johnson, 1803), 531. Rather ironically, Malthus noted in this edition (p. 37): 'Mathematical terms carry with them an imposing air of accuracy and profundity, and ought, therefore, to be applied strictly, and with the greatest caution, or not at all'. For Robert Southey, see above, ref. 2, 135.
20. William Coleman, 'Medicine against Malthus: François Mélier and the Relation Between Subsistence and Mortality (1843)', *Bulletin of the History of Medicine*, liv (1980), 23–43.
21. It should be said here that we lack a detailed study of the politics of the medical profession in England at this time. For some approaches and bibliography see Dorothy Porter and Roy Porter (eds), *Doctors, Politics and Society: Historical Essays* (Amsterdam: Rodopi, 1993).
22. James, *Population Malthus*, 5.
23. Thomas Short, *A General Chronological History of the Air...* (London: Longman and Millar, 1749).
24. For Cobbett see Kenneth Smith, *The Malthusian Controversy* (London: Routledge and Paul, 1951), 120.
25. Christiana C. Hankin (ed.), *Life of Mary Anne Schimmelpenninck*, 2 vols (London: Longman, Brown, Green, Longman's and Roberts. 1858), i, 151–3, cited in Desmond King-Hele, *Doctor of Revolution: The Life and Genius of Erasmus Darwin* (London: Faber & Faber, 1977), 46.
26. Maureen McNeil, *Under the Banner of Science: Erasmus Darwin and His Age* (Manchester: Manchester University Press, 1987), 91; King-Hele, *Doctor of Revolution*.
27. William Hazlitt, *The Spirit of the Age* (Menston, Yorks: Scolar Press, 1971), 251–76.
28. James, *Population Malthus*, 25. On medical and theological materialism, see also Catherine Gallagher, 'The Body Versus the Social Body in the Works of Thomas Malthus and Henry Mayhew',

in Catherine Gallagher and Thomas Laqueur (eds), *The Making of the Modern Body: Sexuality and Society in the Nineteenth Century* (Berkeley: University of California Press, 1987), 83–106; Brian Young, *Religion and Enlightenment in Eighteenth-Century England* (Oxford: Clarendon Press, 1998); A. M. C. Waterman, *Revolution, Economics and Religion: Christian Political Economy, 1793-1833* (Cambridge: Cambridge University Press, 1991).

29. For discussion of Townsend, see Smith, *The Malthusian Controversy*, 28–29.

30. For 'eat or be eaten', see Desmond King-Hele, *The Essential Writings of Erasmus Darwin* (London: MacGibbon and Kee, 1968), 94. On Darwin, see McNeil, *Under the Banner of Science.*

31. On vaccination and its opponents, see G. Miller, *The Adoption of Inoculation for Smallpox in England and France* (London: Oxford University Press, 1957).

32. See Roy Porter, *Doctor of Society: Thomas Beddoes and the Sick Trade in Late Enlightenment England* (London: Routledge, 1991).

33. On Charles Hall see Smith, *The Malthusian Controversy*, 50f.

34. Charles Hall, *The Effects of Civilization on the People in European States* (London: printed for the author, 1805). Some copies contain an Appendix: *Observations on the Principal Conclusion in Mr. Malthus's Essay on Population.*

35. Hall, *The Effects of Civilization*, quoted in Smith, *The Malthusian Controversy*, 51.

36. Hall, quoted in Smith, *The Malthusian Controversy*, 52.

37. Hall, quoted in Smith, *The Malthusian Controversy*, 52.

38. Hall, quoted in Smith, *The Malthusian Controversy*, 53.

39. Hall, quoted in Smith, *The Malthusian Controversy*, 53.

40. Hall, quoted in Smith, *The Malthusian Controversy*, 54.

41. Hall, quoted in Smith, *The Malthusian Controversy*, 55.

42. For Thomas Jarrold (1770-1853), the main sources of information remain the *Dictionary of National Biography* entry, and the discussion in Smith, *The Malthusian Controversy*, 56f. He would repay further study.

43. Thomas Jarrold, *A Letter to Samuel Whitbread, M. P. ... on the Poor's Laws* (London: Cadell and Davis, 1807); *Anthropologia, or Dissertations on the Form and Colour of Man* (London: Cadell and Davis, 1808); *An Inquiry into the Causes of the Curvature of the Spine* (London: Longman, Hirst and Rees, 1823); *Instinct and Reason Philosophically Investigated, With a View to Ascertain the Principles of the Science of Education* (Manchester: Longman, Rees, Orme, Browne and Longman, 1836); *Education of the People* (Manchester:

Longman, Rees, Orme, Browne and Longman, 1847). Jarrold was a member of the Manchester Literary and Philosophical Society, and in 1811 contributed to its *Memoirs* a paper on 'National Character' (2nd series, ii. 328).

44. Jarrold, *Dissertations on Man, Philosophical, Physiological and Political, ... in Answer to Mr. Malthus's Essay on the Principle of Population* (London: Cadell and Davis, 1806).

45. Jarrold, *Dissertations on Man*, 61.

46. Jarrold, *Dissertations on Man*, 20.

47. Jarrold, *Dissertations on Man*, 69.

48. Jarrold, *Dissertations on Man*, 73.

49. Jarrold, *Dissertations on Man*, 267.

50. Jarrold, *Dissertations on Man*, 265, 71.

51. Jarrold, *Dissertations on Man*, 361.

52. Jarrold, *Dissertations on Man*, 250.

53. Jarrold, *Dissertations on Man*, 366.

54. Michael Ryan *The Philosophy of Marriage, in its Social, Moral, and Physical Relations* (London: Baillière, 1843). On Ryan, see Michael Mason, *The Making of Victorian Sexual Attitudes* (Oxford and New York: Oxford University Press, 1994), 185; Roy Porter and Lesley Hall, *The Facts of Life: The Creation of Sexual Knowledge in Britain from 1650 to 1950* (New Haven, Conn.: Yale University Press, 1995), 126.

55. Ryan, *The Philosophy of Marriage*, 13.

56. Ryan, *The Philosophy of Marriage*, 15.
    Much work remains to be done on such figures, one text deserving further study being Henry Thomas Kitchener's *Letters on Marriage, on the Causes of Matrimonial Infidelity, and on the Reciprocal Relations of the Sexes*, 2 vols (London: C. Chapple, Pall Mall, 1812).

57. James, *Population Malthus*, 111–2.

4

'Malthus on Man – In Animals no Moral Restraint'

Robert M. Young

After intensive reflection over several decades I am prepared to announce that there are three and only three possible views about the future: (1) It's definitely going to be okay. (2) It is definitely not going to be okay. (3) It might be okay under certain conditions. These predictions apply variously to the planet, the human species, life on earth, the universe. Condition three has the most variants, some concerning matters outside human control, some up to us. My aim is to explore the question of how anything can be 'up to us' in a Malthusian and Darwinian world of animals, including humans, which obeys deterministic laws. I will suggest that these major figures, in laying the foundations of the social and biological sciences, did provide a space for human praxis. These three positions were also the ones available at the end of the eighteenth century. Condorcet (under sentence of death during the Terror and in hiding) was certain that progress would prevail. William Godwin, whose life was a disaster area which got worse and worse, was equally certain about human perfectibility. Malthus was so clearly sallying forth against their optimism that he said so in the title of the first edition of his polemical tract: *An Essay on the Principle of Population, as it Affects the Future Improvement of Society, with Remarks on the Speculations of Mr. Godwin, M. Condorcet, and Other Writers.* The version of his law in this edition was the clearest and starkest. Food supply could only increase arithmetically, population would increase geometrically. He proposed this as a universal law, valid for all populations at all times.[1]

The imagination is immediately caught by the diverging series of numbers 1, 2, 3, 4, 5, 6, 7, 8, 9 versus 2, 4, 8, 16, 32, 64, 132, 268, 536. On reflection, however, we never experience the higher versions of the ratio, e.g., nine bellyfuls of food available to 536 people. The gap never gets anywhere near that wide because of hunger, starvation, famine, disease, pestilence, death and war. The dynamic of the Malthusian Law is that it is an iron law, and the baleful vicissitudes of human history mathematically demonstrates the brakes on human perfectibility.

Ever since 1798 the name Malthus and the adjective Malthusian have stood for pessimism about what human industry can do in the face of population growth. In fact, as he looked further and further into the matter two crucial modifications came to light. Actual statistics, such as he could discover, were widely varying. Indeed, as subsequent writings, including recent reviews of the literature by Roy Porter and Gertrude Himmelfarb, have shown, the jaws of the crunch between the widening divergence of the ratio do not open anywhere near as wide as his law predicted. Our populations did not grow as fast as he predicted, and our industry is much more effective than he imagined. More importantly, the factor which he called 'moral restraint', a category we would widen from abstinence to include various forms of birth control, produces checks on population growth that he did not imagine possible. We do have all the bad consequences of scarcity which he predicted, but not always or everywhere.

My understanding is that the parameters he laid down are, in the widest sense, the right ones, but there are deeper causes of population growth than he saw. We cannot hope for human good will and felicity to prevail except in a post-scarcity world, but we do not have one, and one is not in sight. In this paper I am going to try to move back and forth between the nineteenth-century understanding of the widest applications of Malthusianism, on the one hand, and more recent renditions of it, on the other. I suggest that we live in the shadow of his formulation and that the terms he propounded for thinking about these matters are undimmed in their appeal, though not, perhaps, in their final usefulness. Indeed, I believe that a suitably expanded modern version of his most derided conceptualisation is perhaps the most useful one.

But first I want to underpin Malthus's significance by connecting his law to Darwinism. Malthus is important to Darwin for three reasons. First, as I never tire of pointing out and certain others never tire of seeking to disprove, Darwin's reading of Malthus in September or October 1838 provided the moment of insight, the key, to the theory of evolution by natural selection. It is basic to Darwinism – a foundation stone for his theory. Second, the tenor, the mood, the rendition of nature which Malthus lent to political economy provided an (I would say *the*) basis for the tone of Darwinism and extrapolations from it which we associated with the struggle for existence, the survival of the fittest, social Darwinism (a theory to which I have argued Darwin adhered[2]) and, in general, with pessimistic notions of nature and human history. Third – and perhaps this should be seen as falling inside my first and second points – The Darwin-Malthus link is the weld which holds together humanity with the rest of living and inorganic nature. I think that bond is why scholars persist in attacking the connection to which I was, I believe, the first to draw attention in a systematic, scholarly way.[3] Marx and Engels and many others did so in a polemical way.

In my opinion Darwin's theory of evolution by natural selection is the most important idea in the history of science, perhaps in the history of thought, as far as the histories of science and of thought centre of the place of humankind in the great scheme of things. I hasten to add that I feel uncomfortable being a bedfellow of some of those who hold this view in ways which overlap with my approach but also diverge from it, e.g., Daniel Dennett and Richard Dawkins. Indeed, Darwin's theory came to replace the deep and pervasive theory which held everything – the cosmos – together from ancient times to the mid-nineteenth century, 'The Great Chain of Being', with its principles of plenitude, continuity and unilinear gradation,[4] beautifully evoked in Epistle II of Alexander Pope's 'Essay on Man' (1733), where we find humanity placed as the middle link in the chain:

> Know then thyself, presume not God to scan;
> The proper study of mankind is Man.
> Plac'd on this isthmus of a middle state,
> A being darkly wise, and rudely great:
> With too much knowledge for the Sceptic side,
> With too much weakness for the Stoic's pride,
> He hangs between; in doubt to act or rest;
> In doubt to deem himself a God, or Beast;
> In doubt his Mind or Body to prefer;
> Born but to die, and reas'ning but to err;
> Alike in ignorance, his reason such,
> Whether he thinks too little, or too much:
> Chaos of Thought and Passion, all confused;
> Still by himself abused, or disabused;
> Created half to rise, and half to fall;
> Great lord of all things, yet a prey to all;
> Sole judge of Truth, in endless Error hurled:
> The glory, jest and riddle of the world![5]

Treating this question of significance somewhat more narrowly, it is said that there have been a number of blows to human arrogance. The concept of the solar system dethroned the Earth from being regarded as the centre of the universe. Darwinism showed that humanity is not the specially created pinnacle of creation. Marxism showed that what humans do is fundamentally conditioned by economic and ideological forces. Freud showed that we do not even have access to the greater part of our motivations, which are unconscious. These explanations mitigate our conception of the human species and our planet as central in the universe and our humanity as characterised by rational intentionality and conscious control over our actions.

If we look at Darwin's theory as one of the great ideas in the history of science, we can characterise it in two ways. Evolution ranks with gravity, the central concept in physics, and affinity, the key idea in chemistry, as one of the most basic concepts in the natural sciences. Beyond that, however, evolution by natural selection is an all-embracing theory in two senses. It is the law which binds all of life together and defines its relations to the physical environment. And, of course, it binds humanity to the rest of life and nature. Evolution by natural selection is the process which accounts for the history of living nature, including human nature.

All of the above is arguably common knowledge. However, there is a huge problem which is left unresolved by evolution. If we take evolution to be an all-embracing explanation of living, including human, phenomena, then it includes human psychology, society and culture within the causal nexus of deterministic scientific laws. If this is so, what is the basis for morality? Put another way, how should we think of the role of values and morality in human nature. At its most stark, evolution by natural selection proceeds by competition for resources for mates to achieve viable offspring which live to reproduce. How can this conception of the interrelations between creatures be subtle enough to include processes which transcend competition – altruism, charity, generosity, including what Malthus called 'moral restraint'? How can it explain the diversity of customs and mores in different cultures? Providing such explanations is, I take it, part of the project of the new Darwinian sciences, in particular Darwinian psychology. The answers they tend to provide often strike me as less useful than the ones we can gain from more traditional ones employing human purposes, consciously conceived and/or discerned in unconscious motivations which do not rely on selfish genes and competition for mates.

It seems to me to be approaching things the wrong way up to

claim that Darwinian explanations provide the most basic accounts for the subtleties and complexities of human relations when literature, philosophy, analytical psychology and other cultural approaches evoke and explore them so well. Perhaps I should say, rather, that it seems wrong-headed to me to offer Darwinian explanations as superior to or as replacements for traditional explorations of such matters in the arts. It may be, of course, that evolution explains humanity and all its works, but we must still find a way of paying due respect to established forms of reflection on human nature and not run headlong into a single explanatory paradigm.

This point becomes an urgent one when science gains access to the mechanisms for altering genetic processes and begins to allow us to reconstruct the genomes and achieve cloning of other species and ourselves. It is too easy to collapse the issues involved and to allow too much authority to scientists in the debates which it is appropriate for us to have about these matters. There is also a common elision which needs to be avoided. It is sometimes thought or implied that since evolution can, in principle, explain everything human, then evolutionists – by which I mean biological scientists – have special insights and authority across all of knowledge. I find this implied in the aggressive stances taken up by some (not all) of the public spokespersons of science. I have in mind, for example, Richard Dawkins and Louis Wolpert, both of whom strike me as delighting in putting down people whose disciplines they assert are made less important and even a waste of time, e.g., philosophy, history and philosophy of science, cultural studies. There was a similar arrogance associated with positivism in earlier decades. There was science on the one hand and confusion on the other; testable hypotheses and muddle, logic and poetry. A whole series of dichotomies was posited with one side reliable and the other markedly less so:

fact-value
science-ideology
nature-culture
science-arts
primary qualities-secondary qualities
mechanism-purpose
outer-inner
rational-emotional

My experience of certain biologists, molecular biologists and scientists who appear on the media and speak in a militant way is that they reproduce the celebration of science at the expense of the rest of knowledge. I advocate complementarity and peaceful coexistence and deplore arrogance. Two examples come to mind. The eminent molecular biologist Sydney (latterly Sir Sydney) Brenner (co-discoverer of the genetic alphabet) was a Fellow of King's College, Cambridge when I was. I invited a distinguished philosopher of science, Mary Hesse, to a college feast, and the person arranging the seating thought it interesting to put them next to each other. When they were introduced and Brenner asked her and was told what her field was, he replied, 'Haven't they wound that up yet?' I told this story in a television debate with Louis Wolpert at a point when he was denigrating scholars whose disciplines involved reflecting on science. His comment was, 'Quite right!'. Aside from the discourtesy to a college guest, I found this insolence characteristic. I have a similar impression from some of the speculations of Richard Dawkins who discusses religion as analogous to a virus and in one article let slip that he regarded culture in the same light. The implied subtext was that scientists might help us root out these infections and leave us with pure scientific rationality. These people may be right to defend themselves against the charge of being reductionists. It is not at all as obvious to me that they are not philistines.

You could be forgiven for beginning to wonder if I have wandered off my topic, but I don't think I have, since I am persuaded that Malthus and the desire to pry him and Darwin apart is central to this debate. Malthus was the only political economist among the authors most cited in Darwin's in his notebooks and early manuscripts and one of the six to be cited ten or more times there as well as in his autobiography.[6] Scientists and their deferential colleagues in the history of science want to keep biology innocent of what they consider to be ideologically-tainted ideas, and Malthus's Law is an excellent example of such a potential pollutant. They want to do this, not because they want to keep clear of matters human but because they want to make extrapolations from biology to the human and social sciences and don't want anyone pointing out that the social and political and ideological conclusions, which they want to claim are pure and legitimate extrapolations from untainted biology, were stuffed into the hat on day one and lie at the foundations of the most basic theory in biology.

But this won't do. I'll now have to go over some old ground in the recent history of the history of science. It is nearly universally acknowledged, as I have said, that I started this hare. I have read several accounts in the course of preparing this paper which say so, e.g., a recent one by Jim Moore and a monograph by Daniel Todes entitled *Darwin without Malthus.* There have been a number of attempts to modify my findings, (one or two arguably Oedipal) by e.g., Bowler, Ghiselin, Mayr, Herbert, Schweber, deBeer. Ingemar Bohlin has even written an admiring but also critical doctoral dissertation on this subject, while a number of others support my position more or less completely, David Kohn, who called my analysis of the Darwin-Malthus link 'nearly definitive', being the most eminent of them.[7] Those who disagree often do so with considerable passion. For example, when I came down to breakfast on the first morning of the conference which led to the publication of *The Darwinian Heritage,* the venerable Ernst Mayr accosted me before I could get some coffee. 'You are Young. You are completely wrong. It is in my book.' Michael Ghiselin was equally cordial and says somewhere 'As a dog returns to its vomit, Robert Young...' I confess to not properly understanding some of the intricacies and minutiae of the attempts to modify or refute my argument about Malthus's role in the origin of Darwin's theory. I find the connection prominent and quite explicit in his notebooks, his pencil sketch of 1842, in his longer sketch of 1844, in the big *Natural Selection* book (of which *On the Origin of Species* was an epitome), in his joint presentation with Wallace, in the structure of the argument of *The Origin,* in his later books, in his correspondence, in his responses to people who ask about this matter, in his agreement with Wallace that he, too, drew inspiration from Malthus[8] and in his autobiography, where he said,

> In October 1838, that is, fifteen months after I had begun my systematic inquiry, I happened to read for amusement Malthus on Population, and being well prepared to appreciate the struggle for existence which everywhere goes on from long-continued observation of the habits of animals and plants, it at once struck me that under these circumstances favourable variations would tend to be preserved, and unfavourable ones to be destroyed. The result of this would be the formation of a new species. Here, then, I had at last got a theory by which to work; but I was so anxious to avoid prejudice, that I determined not for some time to write even the briefest sketch of it.[9]

I am not going to array all this evidence before you; I have done it before.[10] I am going to support it with some new materials and reflections. In preparing this paper I have had recourse to some new sources, in particular, the ten magnificent volumes of Darwin letters which have appeared since 1985. All of this new evidence supports my contentions. For example, there is a letter to Neil Arnott written in February 1869, where Darwin shows that in his own mind his own and Malthus's conceptions are perfectly fused: 'You put the Malthusian *great* truth of the "Struggle for existence" very forcibly'.[11] He elsewhere uses whether or not people share his admiration for Malthus as an acid test of whether or not he considers them intelligent.[12] In one letter to Gray he speaks of a critical review of *The Origin* and concludes: 'The article is a curiosity of unfairness and arrogance. But as he sneers at Malthus, I am content, for it is clear he cannot reason.'[13] In earlier letters he refers to 'Malthus' most logical writings',[14] 'the great Malthus'[15] and 'the great philosopher Malthus'.[16]

I want to reflect on why I have not bothered to check my own research against the points which some of these people have attempted to score against my account of this matter. First, some are patently only interested in separating Darwin from Malthus on the basis of the political belief that it simply cannot be the case that such a pure scientist would pervert objectivity and neutrality with such ideological stuff as Malthus' theory. I see deBeer, Mayr and Ghiselin in this light. But others have looked closely at the details of the elements of Darwin's reasoning, e.g., the difference between inter- and intra-specific competition or how much of a theory had he apparently worked out before October 1838. I suppose I simply have to come clean and say that I don't really care, because I don't think the origins of ideas are that logical or repay that kind of scrutiny. A. O. Lovejoy convinced me long ago that the history of ideas is full of lacunae, inconsistencies, partly worked-out ideas and other sorts of messiness, including eccentric readings of their sources and main influences. We have to take our great thinkers as we find them and not try to shoe-horn them into our own philosophical shoes, as I believe Bohlin, among others, has tried to do. I am a lot more interested in Darwin's account than I am in the perhaps over-zealous scrutiny which leads people to say they know better than he what the precise path, step by step, of his reasoning was, and how he *must have thought* rather than what he says over and over, on the day and repeatedly, about the course of his deliberations.

I want once again to draw attention to what he says about Malthus. I find it exciting and compelling. It jumps out of the page at us and shouts that it provides exactly what he needed, a dynamism, pressure, something to *drive* the process of the origination of new species. In the 1844 Essay, he writes, 'It is the doctrine of Malthus applied in most cases with ten-fold force.'[17] My favourite passage (which gave me my title for this essay) comes from his 1842 pencil sketch of the theory:

> But considering the enormous geometrical power of increase in every organism and as every country, in ordinary cases, must be stocked to full extent, reflection will show that this is the case. Malthus on man – in animals no moral [check] restraint – they breed in time of year when provision most abundant, or season most favourable, every country has its season – calculate robins – oscillating from years of destruction.... the pressure is always ready ... a thousand wedges are being forced into the economy of nature. This requires much reflection; study Malthus and calculate rates of increase and remember the resistance – only periodical.... In the course of a thousand generations infinitesimally small differences must inevitably tell...[18]

Sometime between 28 September and 12 October 1838, he read Malthus (probably his brother's copy). In his Notebook D he wrote (at a later date), 'Towards close I first thought of selection owing to struggle.'[19] Among the pages excised by Darwin for use in writing his great work entitled *Natural Selection*, one finds the following passage:

> [Sept] 28th. We ought to be far from wondering of changes in numbers of species, from small changes in nature of locality. Even the energetic language of Decandolle does not convey the warring of the species as inference from Malthus – increase of brutes must be prevented solely by positive checks, excepting that famine may stop desire. – in nature production does not increase, whilst no check prevail, but the positive check of famine and consequently death. I do not doubt every one till he thinks deeply has assumed that increase of animals exactly proportionate to the number that can live. – . . .

> Population is increase at geometrical ratio in FAR SHORTER time than 25 years – yet until the one sentence of Malthus no one clearly perceived the great check amongst men... The final cause of all this wedging, must be to sort out proper structure, and adapt it to change. – to do that for form, which Malthus shows is the final effect (by means however of volition) of this populousness on the energy of man. One may say there is a force like a hundred thousand wedges trying [to] force every kind of adapted structure into the gaps in the oeconomy of nature, or rather forming gaps by thrusting out weaker ones.[20]

In Notebook E, begun in October 1838, the excitement is

palpable.

He quotes Malthus:

"It accords with the most liberal! spirit of philosophy to believe that no stone can fall, or plant rise, without the immediate agency of the deity [Malthus wrote "divine power"]. But we know from experience! that these operations of what we call nature, have been conducted almost! invariably according to fixed laws: and since the work began, the causes of population & depopulation have been probably as constant as any of the laws of nature with which we are acquainted." – This applies to one species – I would apply it not only to population & depopulation, but extermination and production of new forms – this number and correlations.[21]

So – Darwin sees his theory as a generalization of Malthusianism. On the next page Darwin mentions 'my theory' and the small changes involved in the slow process; subsequent pages mention 'the theory' and 'my theory'.

I return now to the tone and impact of Malthus theory. The *laissez-faire* economist Adam Smith and the natural theologian William Paley had postulated an invisible hand, maintaining a just and harmonious society. Smith even had his own 'Law of Population', whereby population would conveniently rise and fall in response to wage rates. There was for him no limit on the accumulation of wealth, and no problem of population. Indeed, there were fears that population had declined, and its increase was considered an unmitigated good, and if it were to decline, according to Paley, that would be a disaster.[22] There was a lot of speculation: the first census was not taken until 1801.

Malthusian pessimism was complemented by Ricardian economics, which replaced the harmony of the invisible hand with the Iron Law of Wages and postulated endless competition. There was a general trend in social theory: the rule was not harmony but structural contradiction, conflict and competition. The natural urge to be generous was declared misguided, since it would only lead to the birth of more and increasingly impoverished offspring.[23] Parish relief was short-sighted, as was the importing of cheap corn. Only *laissez-faire* (about which she writes at length) would lead to a sustainable and decently paid and housed working population. The starkest proving ground for these stern ideas was Ireland, and although the name Malthus appears nowhere in Cecil Woodham-Smith's account of *The Great Hunger*, the spirit of his doctrine, as well as that of *laissez-faire*, pervades her argument about the government policy which made the Irish Famine far worse than it would otherwise have been.

After he read Malthus, Carlyle called economics 'the dismal science'. Godwin complained that Malthus 'had converted friends of progress into reactionaries by the hundreds'[24] and described Malthus; theory as 'that black and terrible demon that is always ready to stifle the hopes of humanity'.[25] Malthus's biographer says that Bonaparte himself was not considered a greater enemy of his species than Malthus. He was said to have defended small-pox, slavery and child-murder, denounced soup-kitchens, early marriage and parish allowances, 'For thirty years it rained refutations.'[26] Between them, Malthus and Ricardo

> changed the world from an optimistic to a pessimistic one. No longer was it possible to view the universe of mankind as an area in which the natural forces of society would inevitably bring about a better life for everyone. On the contrary, those natural forces which once seemed designed on purpose to bring harmony and peace into the world now seemed malevolent and menacing... Malthus and Ricardo had shown that, left to itself, society would proceed to a kind of barely living hell.[27]

In the Malthusian world preventative checks reduce fertility, while positive checks increase mortality: unwholesome occupations, severe labour, exposure to the seasons, extreme poverty, bad nursing of children, urban conditions, excesses of all kinds, diseases, epidemics, war, plague and famine.[28] In the second, much enlarged edition of 1803, he added a new preventative check, moral restraint from early marriage.[29] Now there were three sets of forces which keep population down to the level of subsistence: moral restraint, vice and misery.[30] He made no allowance for birth control, which he abominated. The laws of nature and the passions of mankind are much more important causes of human misery than human institutions, which Godwin had blamed for human misery.[31] He argued that the Poor Laws should be abolished, and, in the meantime, those benefiting from them should not be better than the worst off of the employed.[32]

If we shift our gaze two centuries onward to the most comprehensive and thoughtful book in the current debate over the future of the earth and its inhabitants, Tom Athanasiou's *Slow Reckoning*, we find it littered with the adjective Malthusian, always conveying a hopelessness, always blaming the poor, always evading the question of just where the poor come from and always masking the structured distribution of rewards and of social location. He writes, '"Surplus population", the notion upon which Malthusianism pivots, is an economic concept masquerading as a biological one, a concept irreducibly bound to fear, social insecurity, loss of place, unemployment, and what linguist Noam Chomsky called the "unmentionable five-letter word" – class'.[33] Indeed, Malthus assures us in the last paragraph of the last edition of his *Essay* that the existing class system will never change.[34] Consider another recent source: in the last volume of his trilogy on social biology, entitled *The Legacy of Malthus,* Allan Chase characterises Malthus as the 'sewer of the seed of scientific racism'[35] and approvingly quotes a characterisation of his *Essay* as 'a propaganda tract favouring certain social arrangements'.[36] Clearly, then, Malthus current place in the firmament is as a whipping boy for liberals and radicals. There is even a web site maintained by conservatives seeking to rehabilitate his reputation.

This is not to say that there is no problem of population. On the contrary, according to Avery,

> the world can be divided into two demographic regions of roughly equal size. In the first, which includes North America, Europe, the former Soviet Union, Australia, New Zealand and Eastern Asia, populations have completed or are completing the demographic transition from the old equilibrium where high birth rates were balanced by a high death rate to a new equilibrium with low birth rates balanced by a low death rate. In the second region, which includes Southeast Asia, Latin America. the Indian subcontinent, the Middle East and Africa, populations seem to be caught in a demographic trap, where high birth rates and low death rates lead to population growth so rapid that the development that could have slowed population growth is impossible.[37]

There seems to be no middle ground. According to present rates of growth, the world's population, which was 2.5 billion in 1959[38] will reach 10 billion by 2050, and many countries are exceeding Malthus' estimate of doubling of population in 25 years.[39] The problem, as I say, is not that population is not growing. The problem is why and what political and economic steps are or are not taken to remove the causes. Demography, biology, environmentalism and politics meet here.

My take on the persistence of the term Malthusianism and its evocation has two facets. One is simply pessimistic, reflecting the ideological invocation of Malthus by elitists and scare-mongers over two centuries. The other facet is even more stark but it is not despondent. It is the implication that human survival, that of other animals and the fate of the planet are matters of praxis, and praxis, the willed, purposive acting according to a thought-out set of intentions in a moral framework, is nothing but the lineal descendant, *mutatis mutandis,* of what Malthus, thinking in terms of the choices of his own culture, called 'moral restraint'. Darwin was able to reach his own theoretical formulation by removing moral restraint from the Malthusian theory: 'in animals, no moral restraint'. This was the essential move, leading to an inescapable determinism in the economy of nature. Notice, however, that he made no objection to the concept of moral restraint as a factor in human populations. Indeed, he devoted chapters four and five of *The Descent of Man* to 'The Moral Sense' and '...Intellectual and Moral Faculties...' Darwin did not think deeply about morality, although he did consider that the moral sense had evolved like other functions of the mind.

I turn now to the conundrum which Darwin's theory bequeathed to biology, anthropology and moral philosophy. As that single sentence signalled in *The Origin*: 'Light will be thrown on the origin of man and his history',[40] and, as Darwin confirmed in *The Descent of Man,* his theory brought humanity into the evolutionary story and the process of natural selection. If there is no moral restraint in animals, and if we are animals, it could follow that 'in man, there is no moral restraint'. But that is not what we believe when we hold conferences on the future of the planet and on population control and on global warming and the other issues which will determine *if there is to be a future.* According to the Worldwatch Institute there are six of them which must be addressed if we are to attain sustainability: stabilising population, shifting to renewable energy, increasing energy efficiency, recycling resources, reforestation and soil conservation.[41] I would add the requirements of care over genetic engineering and over weapons of mass destruction and solving the problems posed by the ozone layer and global warming.

So we come back, once again, to Malthus. He built his argument on the terrain that humans, like other organisms, are subject to natural law.[42] We are subject, that is, to the first natural law laid down by the first professor of economics who was also the first professional social scientist and the founder of scientific demography. Yet he also left us in a pivotal place philosophically with his loophole of moral restraint. He was not optimistic about its likely efficacy. I am not sure I am, either, but it is our only hope, and we are in his debt for mentioning it, even if as an afterthought. It leaves us with a space for restraint, by which I do not mean free will in the pure philosophical sense. Rather, I mean relative freedom from overwhelming constraint; a chance to inhibit blindly following sexual urges by means, for example, of sublimation; freedom to relate sympathetically to other people and other creatures and the world about us. It leaves us with a reflexive feature of human nature with which we can reflect on ourselves while being ourselves, ponder human nature and its constructive and destructive potential while remaining fully human, the products of Darwinian evolution and the severe influences from our economic and social conditions which Malthus characterised.

I have read the first and the sixth editions of Malthus' *Essay* and of Darwin's *On the Origin of Species* with considerable care and find important similarities, especially if I include points made in Darwin's *Descent of Man*. All integrate humanity with the rest of living nature in a framework which treats humans and animals as part of nature. There is a single framework of ideas. Both writers also started with relatively pure theories and, as they revised their works with great care in the light of new information and in order to meet objections, watered down their original positions and admixed them with explanatory factors which were not prominent in their first, more polemical and sketchy, tomes. Darwin allowed space for Lamarckian factors and the direct action of the environment in explaining evolution; Malthus allowed more scope for moral restraint. Their contemporary supporters and subsequent interpreters have tried to hold onto the original, relatively unequivocal, theories.

Throughout this essay I have been concerned to hold Darwin and Malthus together and to acknowledge complexity in explanations. My approach is the opposite of reductionism and oversimplification. On the contrary, I am arguing for an integration of the biological and human sciences which does not hand all of our humanity over to the biologists and sociobiologists and Darwinian psychologists, welcome though their insights certainly are. I am proposing an approach to the study of human nature which includes new versions of the concept of moral restraint and opens itself to drawing on moral discourse from ethics, theology, literature, the theatre, cinema, radio, television and the rest of the arts, without dichotomising life and mind, fact and value, science and culture.

At some point we have to take seriously *what Darwin thought* the role of Malthus was in his thinking. From his most private jottings (carefully excised for inclusion in his big book) and his two sketches (one written lest he die before publishing his findings) and throughout his published work and correspondence, he praises

Malthus and acknowledges a profound admiration and debt. People who object to this connection or who wish to circumscribe its role in the origination of the theory of natural selection are failing to take in the forest while concentrating on certain trees. Thirty years ago I wrote about various readings of Malthus in the nineteenth century – by William Paley, Thomas Chalmers, Darwin, Wallace, Spencer, Marx and Engels. My point was two-fold – the common context of biological and social thought and the fact that scientific and philosophical texts, like the Bible, can be read and made use of in a variety of ways. The use which I wish to make is to draw from the deterministic nexus of Malthus and the Malthusian Darwin the idea that a space nevertheless exists for praxis, the pursuit of morally-framed goals. The future of humankind depends on this, and I am glad that Malthus and Darwin, founders of the modern social and biological sciences, granted its potential efficacy. I would like to express the wish that their heirs in the current debates might be as philosophically liberal-minded and sophisticated.

Did you know that Malthus had a hare lip, corrected by surgery, leaving him strikingly handsome? He also had an uncorrected cleft palate, making him difficult to understand. Both, we are told, were inherited from his great great grandfather. They were his biological inheritance, the refractoriness of nature in his own body, his appearance and his ability to speak and be understood. In spite of these disabilities he won prizes for elocution. Once again, praxis over process, something we can perhaps emulate.

Acknowledgement

I would like to acknowledge the assistance of Anna Mayer of the Cambridge Library Darwin Correspondence Project in my research into Darwin's letters.

References

Bohlin, Ingemar (1995). *Through Malthusian Specs? A Study in the Philosophy of Science Studies, with Specific Reference to the Theory and Ideology of Darwin Historiography.* Ph.D. Dissertation, Department of the Theory of Science, University of Göteborg.

Bowler, Peter J. (1976). 'Malthus, Darwin and the Concept of Struggle', *J. Hist. Ideas* 37: 631-50.

Darwin, Charles R. (1836-44) *Charles Darwin's Notebooks, 1836-1844: Geology, Transmutation, Metaphysical Enquiries.* Transcribed and edited by Paul H. Barrett *et al.* British Museum (Natural History/Cambridge University Press, 1987.

_____ (1874). *The Descent of Man and Selection in Relation to Sex* (1871), 2nd edn Murray.

_____ (1958). "Sketch of 1842" In Darwin and Wallace (1958).

Dawkins, Richard (1976). *The Selfish Gene*. Oxford: Oxford University Press; revised edn, 1989.

_____ (1993). 'Viruses of the Mind', in Bo Dahlbom, ed., *Dennett and His Critics*. Oxford: Blackwell, pp. 13-27.

de Beer, Sir Gavin, ed. (1961-2). "The Origins of Darwin's Ideas on Evolution and Natural Selection." Proceedings of the Royal Society I55 B: 321-38.

_____ (1963). *Charles Darwin*. Nelson.

_____ (1968). "The Darwin Letters at Shrewsbury School" *Notes and Records of the Royal Society* 23: 68-85.

Dennett, Daniel C. (1995). *Darwin's Dangerous Idea: Evolution and the Meanings of Life*. N. Y.: Simon & Schuster; reprinted Harmondsworth: Penguin, 1996.

Ghiselin, M. T. (1969). *The Triumph of Darwinian Method*. Berkeley: University of California Press.

Glass, D. V., ed. (1953). *Introduction to Malthus*. Watts.

Herbert, Sandra (1971). 'Darwin, Malthus and Selection'. *J. Hist. Biol.* 4: 209–17.

_____ (1974, 1977). 'The Place of Man in the Development of Darwin's Theory of Transmutation', Parts I and II. *J. Hist. Biol.* 7: 217–58; 10:155-227.

Himmelfarb, Gertrude (1998). 'The Ghost of Parson Malthus', *Times Litt. Supp.* 23 Jan. 1998, pp. 4–5.

Thomas Robert Malthus (1830). *A Summary View of the Principle of Population*. Reprinted in Glass (1953), pp. 113–81.

_____ (1970). *An Essay on the Principle of Population* (1798) and *A Summary View of the Principle of Population* (1830). Harmondsworth: Penguin.

_____ (1986). *The Works of Thomas Robert Malthus*, 8 vols. William Pickering.

Mayr, Ernst (1982). *The Growth of Biological Thought: Diversity, Evolution, and Inheritance*. Cambridge, Mass.: Harvard University Press.

Moore, James (1997). 'Wallace's Malthusian Moment: The Common Context Revisited', in Bernard Lightman, ed., *Victorian Science in Context*. University of Chicago Press, pp. 290–311.

Ospovat, Dov (1979). 'Darwin after Malthus', *J. Hist. Biol.* 12: 211–30.

_____ (1981). *The Development of Darwin's Theory: Natural History, Natural Theology, and Natural Selection, 1838-1859*. Cambridge: Cambridge University Press.

Porter, Roy (1998). 'Why Mr Fax Git It Wrong', *London Rev. of Books* 5 March, pp. 18–19.

Schweber, Silvan S. (1977). 'The Origin of the Origin Revisited', *J. Hist. Biol.* 10: 229–316.

Smith, Sydney (1960). 'The Origin of "The Origin" as Discerned from Charles Darwin's Notebooks and his Annotations in the Books he read between 1837 and 1842', *Advancement of Sci.* no. 64: 391–401.

Stauffer, R. C., ed. (1975). *Charles Darwin's Natural Selection, Being the Second Part of his Big Species Book Written from 1856 to 1858.* Cambridge: Cambridge University Press.

Woodham-Smith, Cecil (1962). *The Great Hunger: Ireland 1845-9.* Hamish Hamilton; reprinted New English Library, 1970.

Young, Robert M. (1985). *Darwin's Metaphor: Nature's Place in Victorian Culture.* Cambridge: Cambridge University Press.

Notes

1. [Thomas Robert Malthus], *An Essay on the Principle of Population, as it Affects the Future Improvement of Society, with Remarks on the Speculations of Mr. Godwin, M. Condorcet, and Other Writers* (London: J. Johnson, 1798; reprint Ann Arbor: University of Michigan Press, 1959), 4–5, 126–7; Thomas Robert Malthus, *An essay on the Principle of Population; or, a View of Its Past and Present Effects on Human Happiness; an Inquiry into Our Prospects Respecting the Future Removal or Mitigation of the Evils which It Occasions*, 6th edition, 2 vols (London: Murray, 1826), I, 529; John Avery, *Progress, Poverty, and Population: Re-reading Condorcet, Godwin, and Malthus* (London: Cass, 1997), 64.

2. Robert M. Young, 'Darwinism *is* Social', in David Kohn (ed.), *The Darwinian Heritage* (Princeton, N.J.: Princeton University Press, 1985).

3. Robert M. Young, 'Malthus and the Evolutionists: The Common Context of Biological and Social Theory', *Past & Present* 43 (1969), 109–45.

4. Arthor O. Lovejoy, *The Great Chain of Being: A Study of the History of an Idea* (Cambridge, MA: Harvard University Press, 1936; reprinted New York: Harper Torchbooks, 1960).

5. Alexander Pope, 'An Essay on Man' (1733); reprinted in *Poems of Alexander Pope* (Nelson, n.d.), 116–54.

6. Daniel R. Todes, *Darwin without Malthus: The Struggle for Existence in Russian Evolutionary Thought* (New York and Oxford: Oxford University Press, 1989), 125, citing Manier.

7. David Kohn, 'Theories to Work By: Rejected Theories, Reproduction and Darwin's Path to Natural Selection' *Studies in the History of* Biology 4 (1980), 67–170; see also David R. Oldroyd, 'How Did Darwin Arrive at His Theory? The Secondary Literature to 1982' *History of Science* 22 (1984), 325–74.

8. Charles R. Darwin, *The Correspondence of Charles Darwin*, 10 vols (Cambridge: Cambridge University Press, 1985–97), VII, 279.

9. Charles R. Darwin, *The Autobiography of Charles Darwin 1809-1882 with original omissions restored*, Nora Barlow (ed.) (London: Collins, 1958), 120.

10. Young, 'Darwinism *is* Social', 40–44.

11. Darwin, *Correspondence*, VIII, 90.

12. Darwin, *Correspondence*, VIII, 238, 242.

13. Darwin, *Correspondence*, VIII, 247.

14. Darwin, *Correspondence*, V, 416.

15. Darwin, *Correspondence*, II, 423.

16. Darwin, *Correspondence*, VIII, 238.
17. Charles R. Darwin and A.R. Wallace, *Evolution by Natural Selection* (Cambridge: Cambridge University Press, 1958), 116.
18. Darwin and Wallace, *Evolution by Natural Selection*, 46–7.
19. Sir Gavin de Beer (ed.), 'Darwin's Notebooks on Transmutation of Species', Parts 1–5 *Bulletin of the British Museum (Natural History)* Historical Series 2 (1960–1), Part III, 128.
20. De Beer, *et al.*, 'Darwin's Notebooks on Transmutation of Species' (1967).
21. De Beer, 'Darwin's Notebooks on Transmutation', Part IV, 160, quoting Malthus, *Principle of Population* (1826), I, 529.
22. Robert L. Heilbroner, *The Worldly Philosophers. The Lives, Times and Ideas of the Great Economic Thinkers* (New York: Simon & Schuster, 1953), 57–8, 67–70.
23. Malthus, *Principle of Population* (1826), II, chapters 2–7.
24. Heilbroner, *The Worldly Philosophers*, 71.
25. Quoted in Heilbroner, *The Worldly Philosophers*, 76.
26. James Bonar, *Malthus and His Work* (London: Macmillan, 1885), 2.
27. Heilbroner, *The Worldly Philosophers*, 94–5.
28. Avery, *Progress, Poverty and Population*, 65.
29. Malthus, *Principle of Population* (1826), I, 15–16, 15f–17f, 534–5.
30. Malthus, *Principle of Population* (1826), I, 534.
31. Malthus, *Principle of Population* (1826), II, 27–8.
32. Avery, *Progress, Poverty and Population*, 75.
33. Tom Athanasiou, *Slow reckoning: the ecology of a divided planet* (London: Secker & Warburg, 1997).
34. Malthus, *Principle of Population* (1826), II, 441, see also 36.
35. Allen Chase, *The Legacy of Malthus: The Social Costs of the New Scientific Racism* (New York: Knopf, 1977).
36. Chase, *The Legacy of Malthus*, 77.
37. Avery, *Progress, Poverty and Population*, 107.
38. Boulding in Malthus, *Principle of Population* (reprint 1959), vi.
39. Avery, *Progress, Poverty and Population*, xiii.
40. Charles Darwin, *On the Origin of Species by Means of Natural Selection, or the Preservation of Favoured Races in the Struggle for Life* (1859, facsimile reprint New York: Athenaeum, 1967), 488.
41. Avery, *Progress, Poverty and Population*, 115.
42. Todes, *Darwin without Malthus*, 13.

5

Malthus Among the Theologians

Brian Young

The history of political economy in Britain can be interpreted at least as much as a plea for the establishment of an educational programme as it can as the development of a new way of analysing human society. Its institutionalisation in the predominantly clerical universities of late eighteenth- and early nineteenth-century Britain has finally begun to be seriously studied, and the published lecture courses of men such as Richard Whately and his fellow Drummond professors at Oxford have proved a useful source for such study.[1] When affirming an insight of the chief instigator of the academic study of political economy, Malthus adverted to the circumstances which often produced this sometimes unpredictable collusion between clericalism and the development of any new academic discipline: 'It is a just remark of Adam Smith, that the attempts of the legislature to raise the pay of curates had always been ineffectual, on account of the cheap and abundant supply of them, occasioned by the bounties given to young persons educated for the church at the universities.'[2] In such a society, the deeply clerical cast of even the most apparently worldly of sciences was, before the intellectual and religious crises of the mid-nineteenth century began to take their secularising effect, something of an inevitability.[3]

The work of Malthus, himself a sometime curate, at the East India College is clearly part of this educative process, and his own pleas for the teaching of political economy in the *Essay* were plainly deeply felt. Nor yet was this education to be restricted to those members of the upper and middle classes who studied at the universities. Malthus felt that 'a few of the simplest principles of political economy' could be taught to the poor. The benefit of this education to society at large would, he argued, have been 'almost incalculable.'[4] On this matter, Malthus was also following the radical thinking of Gilbert Wakefield, his former tutor at Warrington Academy.[5] Institutionalisation, at whatever level, is not, however, the same as professionalisation, and one has to realise that few political economists could have been described simply as 'political economists' during the period of Malthus's working life.

For all his desires that political economy be taught to working people, Malthus was actually less certain how it might be taught to them than he was thoroughly convinced that it ought to become a subject of university education. The Smithian division of labour was not, however, as applicable to the clerisy employed in the universities as it was to the emerging numbers of factory workers. Hence, in large part, the significant interpretative problem of identifying precisely what it was Malthus saw himself as doing in preparing the various editions of the *Essay*. This problem is made all the more acute because of his status as an Anglican clergyman. Plainly, those who responded to him, either positively or negatively, frequently thought of him as having a dual office as priest and teacher. William Godwin, against whose earlier incarnation as perfectibilist Utopian Malthus had directed so much of the energy of his *Essay*, denounced him in 1820 as the clerical fabricator of an anti-Christian doctrine which required not only a new religion for its effective promulgation, but also a new God.[6] In a miscellaneous tract published in 1838, William Manning, an autodidact Treasury messenger who argued for democracy against the politico-religious 'superstitions' of his time, likewise lamented Malthus's doctrine of population, declaring its author to be 'an enemy of human nature, and his doctrine a tissue of falsehood and impiety towards the Creator and preserver of the universe.'[7] Such lay denunciations emphasised Malthus's clerical office in order further to expose his supposedly anti-Christian sentiments. Malthus could thus be disparaged not only as a hireling to the great, preaching a doctrine which Godwin considered acceptable only to aristocrats and aldermen, but also, and potentially even more damagingly, as a hypocritical priest:[8] hence, perhaps, something of Marx's venomous appraisal of 'Pastor' Malthus, a sobriquet borrowed from Cobbett and approved of by Hazlitt.

Was Malthus necessarily a theologian and a moral philosopher, as well as a political economist? Certainly, no rigid departmentalism prevailed in the late eighteenth and early nineteenth centuries, and it is Malthus as theologian, both implicit and explicit, who will be the focus of this essay. The essay's title has been influenced by Stephen M. Fallon's *Milton among the philosophers* (1991), a fascinating study of a poet who was also necessarily a philosopher, and it is such a sense of the essential permeability of office and purpose that will inform the following discussion of Malthus's *Essay*. In developing this aspect of Malthus's thought, due regard has to be paid to the claim made by

A.M.C. Waterman that Malthus was the founder, and *The Essay* of 1798 the founding text, of what he has called Christian Political Economy, which dominated discussion in this area of moral debate until the Poor Law Amendment Act was instituted in 1834.[9]

In his discussion of political economy as a means of education, Malthus also made much of the role of public moralists which was then regularly assumed by members of the clergy. Characteristically, Malthus made a great deal of their supposed failure in this role. It was their maladroit interventions in what E.P. Thompson famously described as the 'moral economy' which was the immediate cause of Malthus's potentially fratricidal ire, and their double-role as irresponsible instigators and implicit repressors was what he denounced most fiercely:

> During the late dearths, half of the gentlemen and clergymen in this kingdom richly deserved to have been prosecuted for sedition. After inflaming the minds of the common people against the farmers and corn-dealers, by the manner in which they talked of them or preached about them, it was but a feeble antidote to the poison which they had infused coldly to observe that, however the poor might be oppressed or cheated, it was their duty to keep the peace.[10]

At the close of this particularly vituperative note, Malthus observed that 'Political economy is perhaps the only science of which it may be said that ignorance of it is not merely a deprivation of good, but produces great evil.' Here, then, neatly described is Malthus's sense of a moral evil which he was to articulate in the form of a deeply practical theodicy. Political economy may have been a worldly science, but it was also a theological tool with considerable apologetic powers. Malthus's fellow clergy had, he felt, failed to appreciate this; and they would continue to do so. In exploring this essential dimension of Malthus's thought, considerable attention has to be paid to his Cambridge education, a matter of which Waterman has rightly made much.

The institutionalisation of the various schools and styles of theology prevalent in eighteenth- and nineteenth-century Britain is finally being analysed with the precision it deserves. Cambridge had very definite associations with different, sometimes competing, theological schools, and these distinctions were often reducible to the level of the collegiate provenance of different scholars and teachers. King's under Charles Simeon, and Magdalene under Peter Peckard (himself a theological liberal despite an education at orthodox Oxford), were establishing themselves during Malthus's undergraduate years as centres of Evangelical high seriousness. Peterhouse, under the mastership of Edmund Law, a progressive theologian, was enjoying its final glory days as a centre of liberal thought. Malthus's own college, Jesus, was a powerhouse of theological and political radicalism. William Paley, a protégé of Law, and a man who was both to influence and to be influenced by Malthus, had once been offered the mastership of Jesus, but he had turned it down in favour of quiet preferment in Cumberland.[11] It is to the circle dominated by Law, of which Paley was the young star, that attention has to be paid when attempting to understand the theological roots of Malthus's *Essay*.

Edmund Law had been deeply involved in the adjudication of Viscount Townshend's prizes in political economy at Cambridge in the 1750s; significantly, one of the first beneficiaries of the prize was William Bell, a future treasurer of St Paul's, who successfully presented an essay on population in 1756, which was to be translated into German in 1762.[12] Bell's was a strongly conservative argument, his language typical of the clerical critique of luxury dominant throughout the greater part of the eighteenth century. He assumed that the ancient world had contained a larger population than the feebler modern states of Europe. Frugality of taste and simplicity in manners guaranteed increasing populousness, which Bell conventionally assumed to be an unassailable good. Agriculture was therefore to be preferred to the commercial production of mere luxury goods; rustic virtue challenged the debaucheries and lewdness of cities. The indissoluble connection between the dangers of debauchery and the virtues of marriage which later informed so much of Mathus's thinking took a rather different form in Bell: luxurious living obliged the rich to keep servants whose low wages left them unable to marry, so that an increase in celibacy was seen to be a necessary concomitant of purely commercial riches. A nation given up to the dubious arts of luxurious living thus conspired 'to make celibacy a fashionable state, and marriage the general object of ridicule and contempt.'[13] Morality and political economy were thereby enmeshed in Bell's work in ways that were to be challenged by Malthus's altogether less nostalgic arguments.

Edmund Law had himself originally made his name with an annotated translation of the major British theodicy of the early eighteenth century, Archbishop William King's *De origine mali*. In his introduction to this work, Law laid down the value and usefulness of a theodicy:

> I have always look'd upon an Enquiry into the Cause and Origin of
> Evil, as one of the noblest and most important Subjects in Natural
> Theology ... It contemplates the Divine Oeconomy in the
> Government of the Universe, searches into the various Schemes of
> Providence, and takes in the whole Compass of Nature. It concerns
> every Man who pretends to act upon any serious Views here, or to
> entertain any solid Hopes of Futurity.[14]

The creation of a theodicy was a project which linked the work
of Law with that of Paley, and, ultimately, also with that of Malthus.[15]
Plainly, although at very different degrees of involvement, all three
men were also interested in the development of political economy as
a subject of university study. For Law, very much the politically astute
Cambridge Whig, this study was to be stimulated by such externally
induced sources as Viscount Townshend's prizes; Paley included
elements of political economy in the lectures on moral and political
philosophy which he successfully delivered at Cambridge in the
1760s and 1770s, and which were published in 1785 as his *Elements
of Moral and Political Philosophy*. Paley's work was quickly to become
the staple of instruction in these matters at Cambridge, and Malthus
was therefore early exposed to his thinking. As a result of several of
the arguments contained in the *Principles*, Waterman, following John
Maynard Keynes, has gone so far as to nominate Paley to the status
of the first of the Cambridge economists.[16]

It was not, however, merely in the field of political economy that
Malthus was indebted to the Law circle. His metaphysical and
theological thinking, especially as declared in the final two chapters
of the original 1798 edition of the *Essay*, was deeply influenced by
the often deeply contentious speculations encouraged by Law and his
younger followers. It is also to be remembered that Malthus had been
taught by Gilbert Wakefield, a former fellow of Jesus, who had been
obliged to resign from his living in the Church of England as a result
of his open adoption of Unitarian ideas. It was Daniel Malthus's
decision to send his son to his tutor's old college which guaranteed
him a further, more prolonged exposure to such ideas. Law had
himself frequently been accused of being at least tacitly a Socinian;
Leslie Stephen referred to this very particular circumstance of liberal
Cambridge thinking when he declared that Paley's own provenance
was Socinian in all but name.[17]

An insufficiently orthodox view of the Trinity was widely held to
lie behind the Peterhouse-inspired petition against clerical and
undergraduate subscription to the Thirty Nine Articles, which was to

be heavily defeated in a Commons debate on the matter in 1772.[18] Joseph Cornish, a Unitarian, nevertheless felt emboldened in the wake of this severe crisis for liberal theology to publish a pamphlet which incited Law, the bishop of Carlisle, to abandon his supposed compromise with the corrupt theology and baneful hierarchy of the Church of England. Cornish wanted Law to announce an attachment to the new denomination which had been founded in the wake of their parliamentary defeat by two of the bishop's more active protégés, Theophilus Lindsey and John Jebb.[19] Wakefield would later announce his approbation of Paley's lectures in moral and political philosophy, although he condemned the defence of subscriptions which, despite his closeness to Law, the increasingly conservative Paley had also made in the course of that work. Although the older generation of Law and his adjutant Francis Blackburne remained in the Church, alongside the younger Paley, the world championed by Cornish and shaped by Lindsey and Jebb claimed the allegiance of Wakefield and other former Cambridge dons. Their theology frequently merged with that of such Rational Dissenters as Joseph Priestley, once an instructor at the Warrington Academy which employed Wakefield and educated Malthus, and himself an enthusiast for teaching the elements of political economy to the middle classes.[20] Malthus had thus experienced the most radical dimensions of Cambridge theology before even going up to Jesus College.

If heterodoxy concerning the central doctrine of the Trinity could be imputed to the Law circle, so also could allied metaphysical and theological concerns. One such, which can be traced at least implicitly in Malthus's thinking, was the heresy of mortalism, which can be simply defined as the belief that the soul actually slept between the death of the individual person and his or her restoration to life at the General Resurrection. Mortalists, who included Milton among their number, thus denied the intermediate state; the followers of Calvin and other enforcers of Protestant orthodoxy would therefore continue eagerly to denounce mortalists as heretics.[21] There were two sources for the mortalist strain in Law's thought: the Scriptures, and the notorious remarks concerning 'thinking matter' contained in Locke's *Essay Concerning Human Understanding*. The Scriptural authority for the claims promoted by Law were subject to much debate, while Locke's unsettling suggestion had given vent to a lively debate among philosophers and theologians.[22] A strongly materialistic understanding of the nature of human consciousness was thus available for Christian thinkers, since Locke had seen no *a priori* incompatibility between a strongly physical understanding of mind and the creative superintendence of God. Something of a compromise between Locke and orthodox defenders of immaterialism had been attempted by yet another former fellow of Jesus, David Hartley, who had taken up a medical career when his conscience forbade him from subscribing to the Thirty Nine Articles as a clergyman. Hartley's doctrine of nerves, vibrations and the medullary substance had not, however, won him many followers, although Joseph Priestley happily engaged with his work.[23]

Hartley's *Observations on man* (1749) shared a major feature with the concerns of Law and his followers: it was, in major respects, a theodicy, although one grounded in an optimism which Malthus did not ultimately share. Hartley had set himself to study 'the Balance of Happiness or Misery, conferred upon the whole System of sentient Beings, and upon each individual of this great System.' He decreed that 'God will be equally benevolent to each, and infinito-infinitely to the whole system.' Hartley, however, repudiated annihilationism, a heresy which was to be adopted by Malthus, and which may also have been present in Paley's thinking, at least when he was a young man. Hartley could not disguise his contempt for the notion that the souls of the wicked would be annihilated at their deaths, not least since he had strongly presumed that 'The great desire of a future Life, with the Horror of Annihilation, which is observable in a great Part of Mankind, are Presumptions for a future Life, and against Annihilation.'[24]

Unlike Law and several of his other elders, including Hartley, Paley largely managed to avoid inclusion in the numbers of the theologically suspect as calculated by their orthodox enemies. This had not always been so; and it is interesting that his first major brush with the orthodox had concerned a proposition which he had kept for his degree. Paley had wanted to defend the claim that the eternal punishment of the wicked contradicted the Divine attributes, a potentially disastrous assertion in the face of disturbingly active orthodox opposition. He was fortunately saved from this danger by the timely insertion by a concerned and equally liberal Richard Watson of a decisive 'non', so that his proposition safely read, 'Aeternitas poenarum *non* contradicit divinis attributis.'[25] Paley seemed uncertain of what would have become of the wicked after their temporally specific punishments were over.

Other seventeenth- and eighteeenth-century theologians were more certain on this matter. They tended to follow the heresy associated with Origen, who had insisted that the souls of the damned were, mercifully, not to be subject to eternal punishment, but were instead merely to be purged of their sins by a fixed term of punishment, and which were thus to be purified into a state allowing for the universal salvation of all humanity. This was the doctrine of universalism, and it was promoted by Hartley, as well as by the Unitarians who wrote in his wake. A preference arose among some theologians influenced by Origen for the opinion that the souls of the wicked would be annihilated at death, which they considered a more just punishment than either eternal or even limited periods of torment, and one which they also thought to be less morally opprobrious when seeking to reconcile a benevolent God with ethically dubious doctrines of punishment. A prominent spokesman for this view was Newton's heretical successor in the Lucasian chair at Cambridge, William Whiston, whose *The eternity of Hell torments considered* (1740), was the focus of considerable controversy.[26] Whiston's apologetic concern with reconciling God's goodness with humanity's frequently malign state was also a dominant feature of Malthus's work.

Any reading of Malthus would affirm his strongly corporeal interpretation of humanity, from the concern with food supply to the control of sexual instincts. As he rather decorously though no less startlingly stated it, 'After the desire of food, the most powerful and general sense of our desires is the passion between the sexes, taken in an enlarged sense.'[27] It was the avowedly basic nature of his understandings of life and its purposes which so appalled the likes of Manning and other religiously-inclined critics. A reading of his two theologically-orientated closing chapters in the 1798 edition of the *Essay* confirms this decidedly physical analysis of the divine creation. Malthus was explicit in detailing the means of his interpretation of natural religion, and it is one which prepares one for his strongly materialistic bias: 'we should reason from nature up to nature's God, and not presume to reason from God to nature.' Furthermore, he underpins this with a decidedly materialistic observation: 'The first great awakeners of the mind seem to be the wants of the body.' The body and its promptings are so vital to his thinking as even to dictate the nature of his eschatology.[28] This is especially obvious in his remarks on the annihilation of the wicked, where he makes emphatic what Paley had left demurely obscure.

The Lockean notion of 'thinking matter' is plainly a working hypothesis for Malthus, who refuses to make a clear distinction between mind and matter, noting rather the suggestive intimacy of the mind and the body. Indeed, a process was discerned over which God alone had control, and which made sense of this seemingly intractable metaphysical puzzle, at least to Malthus's satisfaction:

> it cannot be inconsistent either with reason or revelation, if it appear
> to be consistent with the phenomena of nature, to suppose that God
> is constantly forming mind out of matter, and that the various
> impressions that man receives through life, is the process for that
> purpose.

If Locke's influence is to be inferred here, it is made explicit in
Malthus's assumption that the evil present in the world was necessary
for the mind to continue creating itself through moral and mental
exertion. This was a process to be discerned by different judges who
would come together to accept its lessons, a division of physical and
intellectual labour to which Malthus the political economist
implicitly contributes his share in the great task of understanding
that is the basis of a Newton-inspired natural religion:

> The constancy of the laws of nature, is the foundation of the
> industry and foresight of the husbandman; the skilful researches of
> the physician, and anatomist; and the watchful observation and
> patient investigation of the natural philosopher. To this constancy,
> we owe all the greatest, and noblest efforts of intellect. To this
> constancy, we owe the immortal mind of a Newton.

Theodicy and eschatology necessarily inform each other in
Malthus's ready dismissal of the roles of the wicked in both life and
death:

> The greatest talents have been frequently misapplied, and have
> produced evil proportionate to the extent of their powers. Both
> reason and revelation seem to assure us, that such minds will be
> condemned to eternal death; but while on earth, these vicious
> instruments performed their part in the great mass of impressions,
> by the disgust and abhorrence which they excited.

The 'Scriptural denunciations of eternal punishment', themselves
'a vast and gloomy idea', had not impressed themselves thoroughly on
humanity; and this was a good thing, since if they had done so moral
conduct would have been valueless, conducted solely as it would have
been on a fear of punishment and an expectation of reward. Virtue
resided in love, not in fear; God would not therefore enforce eternal
suffering as a means of eliciting virtue from his creation. The 'Light
of the gospel' had revealed that righteousness led to eternal life, and
that the wages of sin were quite literally to be interpreted as death.
The 'misshapen' wicked would thus 'mix again with their original

clay.' There is a definite echo of Paley's undergraduate proposition in Malthus's conclusion that:

> The Supreme Being would appear to us in a very different view, if we were to consider him as pursuing the creatures that had offended him with eternal hate and torture, instead of merely condemning to their original insensibility those beings, that, by the operation of general laws, had not been formed with qualities suited to a purer state of happiness.[29]

It was primarily Malthus's predilection for the annihilationist hypothesis that would lead him, at the prompting of friends, to remove the explicitly theological closing chapters from future editions of the *Essay*. A letter from a Jesus colleague, Edward Daniel Clarke, had informed Malthus of the reactions to his work of two other clerical fellows of the college, Thomas Cautley and Thomas Castley, as elicited in conversation with a fourth man, Bridge of Peterhouse. Bridge opined that Malthus had unfortunately given grounds to his readers for assuming him to be both a materialist and an annihilationist, though Bridge himself, intriguingly, believed him to be neither. Clarke defended Malthus's exposition of the doctrine of annihilationism as being perfectly compatible with Scripture, a proposition strongly denied by Cautley and Castley, both of whom stated, citing the relevant biblical texts, that the flesh of the resurrected body would answer for 'the Sin committed in the Flesh.'[30] The arguments that had been deployed by orthodox theologians against the mortalism of Law and Blackburne in the 1750s and 1760s were used once more against Malthus's defence of annihilationist doctrine in the 1790s.

Annihilationism would, its opponents supposed, on principles directly contrary to those evinced by Malthus, have dangerously undermined morality by countering one of its great Scriptural and dogmatic guarantees. James Hervey's popular work, *Meditations among the tombs* (1746), had declared for such a view, noting of the fate of the wicked that 'Resurrection will be no Privilege to them, but *Immortality* itself their *everlasting Curse*.' Edward Young's hugely popular *Night Thoughts* likewise contained lines that could easily have been used to contest Malthus's view of the true grounds for living a virtuous life (Night VIII, ll. 1368-69):

> Our Schemes to plan by This World, or the Next
> Is the sole Diff'rence between Wise, and Fool.

In a sermon published in 1743, the Oxford theologian Jeremiah

Seed had identified modern defenders of Origen's proposition as the source of potential moral collapse, requesting that they seriously reflect on the fact that their views gave comfort to the 'Overflowings of Ungodliness.'[31]

By continuing such fraught and inherently dangerous speculations into the 1790s, Malthus was exposing himself to just such accusations from his own contemporaries. Mortality and morality were indissolubly connected for theologians, and Malthus was explicitly challenging a central element in such a moralising eschatology. Furthermore, Malthus had opened up even greater potential for controversy by opining, very much against the theological grain of the eighteenth century, that 'Life is, generally speaking, a blessing independent of a future state.'[32] For some this would have been tantamount to a secular doctrine, as was his equally atypical assumption that life on earth was not to be seen as a 'state of trial' for the next life, which was itself a central dogma of eighteenth-century eschatology, forming the crux of as apologetically important a work as Joseph Butler's *Analogy of religion, natural and revealed* (1736). Edmund Law had also sided with the orthodox on this matter; this life was very much a state of probation in his work, however much his adoption of mortalism might have been seen to contradict this by his consciously orthodox opponents. When Malthus came to abandon these explicitly heterodox theological chapters, he was implicitly to adopt a notion of the connection between morality and mortality which chimed with the utilitarian nature of more orthodox eschatology.[33]

Waterman has argued that Malthus owed much of his heterodoxy in theology to Abraham Tucker, like the Malthus family a comfortable resident of Surrey, and also the eccentric author of a system of natural theology, *The light of nature pursued* (1768-78). This was not so true, however, of Tucker's eschatology which, though odd, was not as obviously heterodox as that proposed by Malthus. Tucker contested Locke's 'thinking matter' hypothesis, preferring to define the mind somewhat ambiguously as 'what is commonly called the human soul.' He also developed a decidedly peculiar eschatology, replete with a notion of the 'vehicular' soul which went on to learn more about the truths of the universe in a surreal version of the intermediate state. Denying the annihilationist hypothesis, Tucker nevertheless questioned the eternal duration of punishments, noting, in a manner reversed by Malthus in 1798, that self-interest dictated one's response to the injunctions of eternity.[34]

Where Tucker does seem to have influenced Malthus was in the notion that God created the world for the formation of mind out of otherwise sluggish matter, observing a progressive struggle between mind and a material world. This in turn may be seen as a theory of mind analogous and complementary to the theory of religious and moral progress which informed the work of Edmund Law and other eighteenth-century theological progressives. Law's theological defences of struggle and his firmly moral encomia to the virtue of work over the vice of idleness presage much in Malthus's *Essay*. For Law, labour restrained man from folly and wickedness, instead improving him in mind and body. Competitive struggle in the world of work and status was likewise divinely beneficial, since:

> Upon this Plan only could there be place for Hope or Fear, Reward or Punishment, the only proper means of governing free, rational Agents, and of conducting them to their supreme and truest Happiness, which seems entirely to consist in Agency, and which can only this way be excited. This therefore is the method most agreeable to Wisdom and Goodness, and consequently most worthy of God.[35]

This had become a theological commonplace by the time that Malthus had integrated it into his theodicy; the semi-utilitarian concern with happiness common to Law and Malthus is also deeply theological in tone, and it is to be remembered that Law's translation of King's theodicy was itself accompanied by an essay by another Cambridge theologian, John Gay, which had developed an early form of theological utilitarianism. There is then, no inherent reason for associating such a deeply religious brand of utilitarianism with an implicitly secularising tendency in either Malthus's thought or in that of his Cambridge predecessors.[36] Theological utilitarianism would maintain an important position in Cambridge until the 1830s, when William Whewell and others moved against what they considered to be its unacceptable degree of psychological hedonism: Malthus's own work would also move some way from such an account, as he emphasised the role of evil in the social order rather less optimistically than had Law and Gay; Malthus sought to explicate 'those deep-seated causes of evil' which resulted from 'the laws of nature.'[37]

Much of Malthus's *Essay* takes the form of extending this theodicy; he ruminates on the connection between 'divine power' and 'fixed laws' in an attempt to understand 'The great plan of providence.' This understanding sometimes involved him in asserting the superiority of apparently worldly reasoning over apparently purely Scriptural reasoning. This is clear in his dismissal of the argument for the common use of property which Godwin, utilising his training as a Dissenting minister, could easily have related to apostolic teaching in the Book of Acts. Despite its advocacy by the Moravians and, for a short time, John Wesley, Malthus insisted that such an institution would serve only to undermine society, not least by its analogous effect on the 'commerce of the sexes.' Security of property and the institution of marriage were the 'two fundamental laws of society', and the common use of property would lay siege to both. In Malthus' view, 'the encouragement and motive to moral restraint are at once destroyed in a system of equality and community of goods.' Malthus's controversial belief in the supreme virtue of 'moral restraint', defined as 'the restraint from marriage which is not followed by irregular gratifications', and which acted as 'the most powerful of the checks' on population, necessarily coalesced for him in a reading of Christian doctrine which neatly combined with the better elements of 'heathen' prudence. Chastity was a virtue common to Christians and the better sort of Roman moralists, but Christianity was supremely and progressively correct on this central matter, since:

> It is a pleasing confirmation of the truth and divinity of the Christian religion, and of its being adapted to a more improved state of human society, that it places our duties respecting marriage and the procreation of children in a different light from that in which they were before beheld.[38]

However consistent with Christian teaching though Malthus found his notion of 'moral restraint', this was an element in his work which generated much criticism on the part of his religious critics. In order to appreciate just how misguided elements of this criticism proved to be, it is well to bear in mind Malthus's claim that, far from maintaining the superior calling of perpetual celibacy, he was in fact reinforcing marriage in the best ways imaginable, not least by providing a strong incitement to industry and the creation of self-worth:

> It is clearly the duty of each individual not to marry till he has a prospect of supporting his children; but it is at the same time to be wished that he should retain undiminished his desire of marriage, in order that he may exert himself to realize this prospect, and be stimulated to make provision for the support of greater numbers.[39]

Misundertandings on this score would persist, however, until they were reified into the arguments of such influential works as

Byron's *Don Juan*, in which Malthus was dismissed with a suitably cavalier disregard for the nuances of his doctrine (Canto XIV, stanzas 37 to 38):

> But Rapp's the reverse of zealous matrons,
> Who favour, malgré Malthus, generation -
> Professors of that genial art, and patrons
> Of all the modest part of propagation,
> Which after all at such a desperate rate runs,
> That half its produce tends to emigration,
> That sad result of passions and potatoes -
> Two weeds which pose our economic Catos.
> Had Adeline read Malthus? I can't tell;
> I wish she had: his book's eleventh commandment,
> Which says, 'thou shalt not marry,' unless well:
> This he (as far as I can understand) meant:
> 'Tis not my purpose on his views to dwell,
> Nor canvass what 'so eminent a hand' meant;
> But certes it conducts to lives ascetic,
> Or turning marriage into arithmetic.

Such was Malthus's concern to see off potential critics of his stance that he sought to preempt the use of the injunction to multiply in Genesis which they predictably went on to make. The dangers of overpopulation were, Malthus insisted, such as to make the Biblical injunction subject to a major worldly qualification: 'A common man, who has read his Bible, must be convinced that a command given to a rational being by a merciful God cannot be interpreted as to produce only disease and death instead of multiplication.'[40] John Young, an Edinburgh solicitor who published under the alias of Simplex, and the veteran of a portmanteau assault on Gibbon, Priestley and Lindsey, expressed his astonishment at Malthus's clerical status when denouncing him in a tract published in 1808. Nor was his sense of astonishment abated as he tore into the doctrine of 'moral restraint': '"MORAL *restraint*," said I, when I first read the phrase! "Paul characterized *forbidding* to marry, the *doctrine of devils*." Methinks, therefore, to any Christian, the word *diabolical*, or *infernal*, would have appeared a much more appropriate epithet than *moral*.' Malthus was, Young continued, contradicting the teaching of Christ and the New Testament as well as undermining the injunction to multiply in Genesis; he was also extolling in celibacy something which had 'a direct tendency to seduction, debauchery, and all manner of uncleanness.' By championing celibacy, albeit of a decidedly temporal sort, Malthus had inadvertently resorted to one of the principal bugbears of British Protestantism, which saw in celibacy remnants of 'Popery' and an enormous potential for sexual perversion.[41]

Young was unhappy at the pessimism which he saw underpinning Malthus's account, regretting that 'this modern reformer' should renounce older ways of appreciating the divine economy: 'Dame Nature was, in days of ancient times, celebrated and extolled for her unbounded munificence, kindness, and indulgence to ungrateful short-sighted mortals. But our author has discovered that she is *harsh* and *cruel.*' Such a renunciation brought with it ill-considered palliatives; temporary celibacy could only lead to pollution and debauchery, promoting a society which would combine the sensual horrors of Sodom and Gommorah with the sin of Onan, that hardy perennial of eighteenth-century purity campaigners, from Tissot and Wesley onwards.[42] Even more disappointingly for Malthus, Richard Watson, a stalwart of Cambridge liberalism, also denounced his views on celibacy, and he did so while brazenly admitting not to have read the *Essay*.

In his memoirs, published in 1817, Watson recalled having received in December 1807 a letter from a clergyman in Bath, who referred flatteringly to Watson's replies to Gibbon and Paine. The clergyman requested that Watson undertake a similar mission in replying to Malthus's *Essay*, which endeavoured, in his opinion, to 'establish a code of morality in opposition to the morality of the Gospel.' As a systematic attack on benevolence he also considered it an affront to the poor (to whom Watson had addressed some rather placatory remarks in 1798, which led in turn to an altercation with Wakefield, an exchange in which Malthus would add his mite, largely on Wakefield's side, in a later edition of the *Essay*). In his reply, Watson accepted that his correspondent's fear regarding the mischief to morals and religions contained in a book which he had not himself read was probably just, concluding with magisterial disdain, that:

> I thought myself justified in thus neglecting to peruse a book thwarting
> the strongest propensity of human nature, and contradicting the most
> express command of God, "Increase and multiply;" especially as I was
> persuaded that the earth had not in the course of six thousand years
> from the creation ever been replenished with any thing like one half of
> the number of inhabitants it would sustain.[43]

Watson's repudiation of Malthus on this point had been matched by Paley's acceptance of the dangerous relationship between the rise of population with the rise in the price of foodstuffs in his *Natural Theology*, published in 1802, some five years before Watson's correspondence with the agitated Bath clergyman. Nor yet was it only amongst the remnants of Cambridge liberalism that Malthus's thesis would be debated; its most consistent adherent came from Simeon's Evangelical King's College: John Bird Sumner, then a master at Eton, produced a study of population and related questions in his own, Evangelical version of a natural theology in 1816.[44] It would, indeed, be largely among the Evangelicals, agitated by the economic questions which arose in the wake of the Napoleonic wars, that Malthus's doctrine would be most seriously considered and most assiduously adopted. Thomas Chalmers, a natural theologian in the style of Paley and Sumner, though with a theology much closer to that of the latter than that of the former, would prove an enthusiastic proponent of Malthus's views.[45]

Malthus, a clerical political economist reared in the closing decades of Cambridge liberalism, would thus continue to inform the practical theology of those very Evangelicals who had reacted so strongly against the sort of liberalism which he had taken to its natural limits in the closing chapters of the first edition of his *Essay*. In this sense, as in so many others, he can be seen as a mediating, perhaps even a transitional figure in the politico-theology conducted in Britain between the French Revolution and the passing of the Great Reform Bill.[46] Although he was, in many ways, a natural radical, his ideas affected the conservative mind rather more than those of his more radical contemporaries; although he was a theological liberal, his legacy was most richly developed by Evangelicals. There is, then, more than a touch of the paradoxical about Malthus and his influence.

Notes

1. Richard Brent, 'God's providence: liberal political economy as natural theology at Oxford, 1825-62' in Michael Bentley (ed.), *Public and Private Doctrine: Essays in Honour of Maurice Cowling* (Cambridge: Cambridge University Press, 1993), 85-107. I am grateful to Donald Winch for his reassuringly supportive reading of my reading of Malthus.
2. Robert Malthus, *An Essay on the Principle of Population*, Donald Winch (ed.) (Cambridge: Cambridge University Press, 1992), 117.
3. B.W. Young, 'Christianity, Commerce and the Canon: Josiah Tucker and Richard Woodward on Political Economy', *History of European Ideas* 22 (1996), 385-400; B.W. Young, 'Christianity, Secularisation and Political Economy' in David J. Jeremy (ed.), *Religion, Business*

    and Wealth in Modern Britain (1998), 35–54.

4. Malthus, *Essay*, 275 and n10.

5. Gilbert Wakefield, *Memoirs of the Life of Gilbert Wakefield* (1804), vol. 1, 363.

6. William Godwin, *Of Population* (1820), 623–24.

7. William Manning, *The Wrongs of Man Exemplified* (1838), 286.

8. Godwin, *Of Population*, 547–48, 565.

9. A.M.C. Waterman, *Revolution, Economics and Religion: Christian Political Economy, 1798–1833* (Cambridge: Cambridge University Press, 1991).

10. Malthus, *Essay*, 275, 10f. For Thompson's critique of Malthus in this regard, see 'The moral economy reviewed' in *Customs in Common* (1991; London: Penguin, 1993), 259–351, at 276, 281–82, 287, 296. Thompson made much of his supposed impact on the future administration of famine relief in India.

11. John Gascoigne, *Cambridge in the Age of the Enlightenment: Science, Religion and Politics from the Restoration to the French Revolution* (Cambridge: Cambridge University Press 1989); Waterman, 'A Cambridge *via media* in late Georgian Anglicanism', *Journal of Ecclesiastical History* 42 (1991), 419–36; J.D. Walsh, 'The Magdalene Evangelicals', *Church Quarterly Review* 159 (1959), 499–511; Charles Smyth, *Simeon and Church Order* (Cambridge: Cambridge University Press, 1940); M.L. Clarke, *Paley: Evidences for the Man* (Toronto: University of Toronto Press, 1974), 42.

12. J.R. Raven, 'Viscount Townshend and the Cambridge Prize for Trade Theory, 1754-1756', *Historical Journal* 28 (1985), 535–55.

13. William Bell, *A Dissertation on What Causes Principally Contribute to Render a Nation Populous, and What Effect has Populousness of a Nation on its Trade* (Cambridge, 1756), 2–3, 5, 8, 13, 18, 22, 24. On the 'luxury debate', see John Sekora, *Luxury: the Concept in Western Thought, Eden to Smollett* (Baltimore and London: Johns Hopkins University Press, 1977), and Christopher J. Berry, *The Idea of Luxury: A Conceptual and Historical Investigation* (Cambridge: Cambridge University Press, 1994), especially chapter 6.

14. 'The translator's preface' to William King, edited and translated by Edmund Law, *An Essay on the Origin of Evil* (1731), iii.

15. Waterman, *Revolution, Economics and Religion*, 126–33.

16. Waterman, 'Why William Paley was "the first of the Cambridge economists"', *Cambridge Journal of Economics* 20 (1996), 673–86; *Revolution, Economics and Religion*, 121.

17. Leslie Stephen, *History of English Thought in the Eighteenth Century*, (1876), vol. 1, 426; G.A. Cole, 'Doctrine, dissent, and the decline of

Paley's reputation, 1805-1825', *Enlightenment and Dissent* 6 (1987), 19–30. For reassessments of Paley's position, see Graham Cole, 'A note on Paley and his school – was Sir Leslie Stephen mistaken?', *Tyndale Bulletin* 38 (1987), 151–56; Neil Hitchin, 'Probability and the Word of God: William Paley's Anglican method and the defense of the scriptures', *Anglican Theological Review* 77 (1995), 392–407; John T. Baldwin, 'God and the World: William Paley's argument from perfection tradition – a continuing influence', *Harvard Theological Review* 85 (1992), 109–20.

18. For discussion, see B.W. Young, *Religion and Enlightenment in Eighteenth-century England: Theological Debate from Locke to Burke* (Oxford: Oxford University Press, 1998), ch. 2.

19. Joseph Cornish, *A Letter to the Right Reverend the Lord Bishop of Carlisle* (1777).

20. Wakefield, *Memoirs*, vol. 1, 116, 129; John Gascoigne, 'Anglican latitudinarianism, Rational Dissent and Political Radicalism in the Late Eighteenth Century', and Alan Tapper, 'Priestley on Politics, Progress and Moral Theology', in Knud Haakonssen (ed.), *Enlightenment and Religion: Rational Dissent in Eighteenth-century Britain* (Cambridge: Cambridge University Press, 1996), 219–40, 272–86.

21. Norman T. Burns, *Christian Mortalism from Tyndale to Milton* (Cambridge, MA: Harvard University Press, 1972); B.W. Young, 'The "Soul-Sleeping System": Politics and Heresy in Eighteenth-century England', *Journal of Ecclesiastical History* 45 (1994), 64–81; Stephen M. Fallon, *Milton Among the Philosophers: Poetry and Materialism in Seventeenth-century England* (Ithaca: Cornell University Press, 1991), 80, 101–10, 129–30.

22. John Locke, *An Essay Concerning Human Understanding*, (ed.) Peter H. Nidditch (Oxford: Clarendon Press, 1975), Book IV, chapter iii; Edmund Law, 'Discourse on the Nature and State of Death'; 'Appendix: Concerning the Use of the Word Soul in Holy Scripture'; 'Postscript': appended to *Considerations on the State of the World with Regard to the Theory of Religion*, (6th edition, Cambridge, 1774), 341–66, 367–435, 437–44. These appendices first appeared in the third edition of the work in 1755. Law did not, though, seem to accept the viability of thinking matter: *An Essay on the Origin of Evil*, 92. For a useful discussion, see John W. Yolton, *Thinking Matter: Materialism in Eighteenth-century Britain* (Oxford: Blackwell, 1984).

23. For an encomium on Hartley both as a former fellow of Jesus and as a critic of the Church of England from an identically placed admirer, see Wakefield, *Memoirs*, vol. 1, 75–8.

24. David Hartley, *Observations on Man, his Frame, his Duty, and his Expectations* (1749), vol. 2, 14, 21, 52, 385, 419–25.

25. Cited in D.L. Le Mahieu, *The Mind of William Paley: A Philosopher and his Age* (London: University of Nebraska Press, 1976), 7–8.

26. D. Walker, *The Decline of Hell: Seventeenth-century Discussions of Eternal Torment* (London: Routledge & Kegan Paul, 1964); Piero Camporesi, *The Fear of Hell: Images of Damnation and Eternal Punishment in Early Modern Europe*, trans. Lucinda Byatt (Oxford: Polity, 1991); Philip C. Almond, *Heaven and Hell in Enlightenment England* (Cambridge: Cambridge University Press, 1994); Paul C. Davies, 'The Debate on Eternal Punishment in Late Seventeenth- and Eighteenth-century English Literature', *Eighteenth-Century Studies* 4 (1970–1), 257–76; Origen, *On First principles* (*De principiis*), trans. G.W. Butterworth (New York: Harper, 1966), 146; Henry Chadwick, 'Origen, Celsus, and the Resurrection of the Body', *Harvard Theological Review* 41 (1948), 83–102; Chadwick, *Early Christian Thought and the Classical Tradition: Studies in Justin, Clement and Origen* (Oxford: Clarendon, 1966), 118–19; Hartley, *Observations on Man*, vol. 2, 419–37; Geoffrey Rowell, 'The Origins and History of Universalist Societies in Britain, 1750-1850', *Journal of Ecclesiastical History* 22 (1971), 35–51.

27. Malthus, *Essay*, 211.

28. Malthus, *First Essay on Population 1798*, J. Bonar (ed.) (London: Macmillan, 1928), 350, 356.

29. *Ibid.*, 354–55, 360–63, 374–75, 386–90.

30. Edward Daniel Clarke to Malthus, August 20th 1798, in J.M. Pullen and Trevor Hughes Parry (eds), *Thomas Robert Malthus: The Unpublished Papers in the Collection of Kanto Gakuen University* (Cambridge: Cambridge University Press, 1998), vol. 1, 73–7.

31. James Hervey, *Meditations Among the Tombs* (1746), 80; Jeremiah Seed, *Discourses on Several Important Subjects* (1743), 93–126.

32. Malthus, *First Essay*, 391.

33. Law, *An Essay on the Origin of Evil*, 273, 307; J.M. Pullen, 'Malthus' Theological Ideas and their Influence on his Principle of Population', *History of Political Economy* 13 (1981), 39–54; Salim Rashid, 'Malthus' Theology: An Overlooked Letter and Some Comments', *History of Political Economy* 16 (1984), 135–38; M.B. Harvey-Phillips, 'Malthus' Theodicy: The Intellectual Background of his Contribution to Political Economy', *History of Political Economy* 16 (1984), 591–608; Samuel M. Levin, 'Malthus and the Idea of Progress', *Journal of the History of Ideas* 27 (1966), 92–108.

34. Waterman, *Revolution, Economics and Religion*, 100–06; Abraham

Tucker, *The Light of Nature Pursued* (1768-78), vol. 2 (part I), 79–80, 117, (part II), 12–335, 457–90.

35. Ronald S. Crane, 'Anglican Apologetics and the Idea of Progress, 1699-1745', *Modern Philology* 31 (1933–4), 273–306, 349–82; Owen Chadwick, *From Bossuet to Newman* (2nd edn., Cambridge: Cambridge University Press, 1987); David Spadafora, *The Idea of Progress in Eighteenth-century Britain* (New Haven, Conn.: Yale University Press, 1990); Law, *Essay on the Origin of Evil*, 124; Law, *Considerations on the State of the World with Regard to the Theory of Religion* (Cambridge, 1745), 17–18.

36. John Gay, *Preliminary Discourse Concerning the Fundamental Principle of Virtue or Morality*, prefaced to Law, *An Essay on the Origin of Evil*. For a rather different view of this matter, see Eric K. Heavner, 'Malthus and the Secularization of Political Ideology', *History of Political Thought* 17 (1996), 408–30. For a succinct statement of the inherently religious dimension of Malthus's thought, see Donald Winch, 'Robert Malthus: Christian Moral Scientist, Arch-demoralizer or Implicit Secular Utilitarian?', *Utilitas* 5 (1993), 239–53.

37. Jacob Viner, *The Role of Providence in the Social Order: An Essay in Intellectual History* (Philadelphia, PA: American Philosophical Society, 1972), 70–5; Malthus, *Essay*, 57.

38. Malthus, *Essay* 40, 86, 604, 77–8, 23, 43–4, 218–19, 221, 223. On Christian use of the argument, see John Walsh, 'John Wesley and the Community of Goods' in Keith Robbins (ed.), *Protestant Evangelicalism: Britain, Ireland, Germany, and America c.1750-c.1950* (Oxford: Basil Blackwell, 1990), 25–50. Malthus' critique echoed that made by Gibbon, who also referred to Plato and More in his denunciation of the doctrine: Edward Gibbon, *The Decline and Fall of the Roman Empire*, (ed.) David Womersley (London: Penguin, 1994), vol. 1, 490, n. 128. More generally, see Neville Morley, 'Political Economy and Classical Antiquity', *Journal of the History of Ideas* 59 (1998), 95–114.

39. Malthus, *Essay*, 215.

40. *Ibid.*, 121.

41. [John Young], *An Inquiry into the Constitution, Government, and Practices of the Church of Christ, Planted by his Apostles* (Edinburgh, 1808), 204–11; B.W. Young, 'The Anglican Origins of Newman's Celibacy', *Church History* 65 (1996), 15–27.

42. Young, *An Inquiry*, 221–22, 229, 231; Thomas Lacqueur, *Making Sex: Body and Gender from the Greeks to Freud* (Cambridge, MA: Harvard University Press, 1990), 227–30.

43. Richard Watson, *Anecdotes of the Life of Richard Watson* (1817), 475-78; Watson, *An Address to the People of Great Britain* (1798); Wakefield, *A Reply to Some Parts of the Bishop of Landaff's Address to the People of Great Britain* (1798); Malthus, *Essay*, 224. Watson claimed to have done what he could for Wakefield when his sometime adversary appealed to him against his imprisonment for the anti-government sentiments contained in his *Reply. Anecdotes*, 305-6. On the strongly counter-revolutionary nature of Watson's *Address*, see Robert Hole, *Pulpits, Politics and Public order in England 1760-1832* (Cambridge: Cambridge University Press, 1989), 152, and on Wakefield's trial, see F.K. Prochaska, 'English State Trials in the 1790s: A Case Study', *Journal of British Studies* 13 (1973), 63–82.

44. William Paley, *Natural Theology* (1802), 539-41; D.L. LeMahieu, 'Malthus and the Theology of Scarcity', *Journal of the History of Ideas* 40 (1979), 467-76; Waterman, *Revolution, Economics and Religion*, 113-70; John Bird Sumner, *A Treatise on the Records of the Creation, and on the Moral Attributes of the Creator; with Particular Reference to the Jewish History, and to the Consistency of the Principle of Population with the Wisdom and Goodness of the Deity*, 2 vols (1816).

45. Boyd Hilton, *The Age of Atonement: The Influence of Evangelicalism on Social and Economic Thought 1785-1865* (Oxford: Oxford University Press, 1988); Waterman, *Revolution, Economics and Religion*, chapter 6.

46. For a thorough appreciation of the subtleties of Malthus's thought, see Donald Winch, *Riches and Poverty: An Intellectual History of Political Economy in Britain, 1750-1834* (Cambridge: Cambridge University Press, 1996), 221–405.

6

Malthus and the Doctors:
Political Economy, Medicine, and the State in England,
Ireland, and Scotland, 1800-1840

Christopher Hamlin and Kathleen Gallagher-Kamper

Curiously, medical history has found little room for Thomas Malthus. Equally curiously, Malthus scholarship has found little room the concepts of health and disease that figure centrally in his work.[1] Yet we know that high levels of deprivation and inequality, sometimes tied to disequilibrium conditions between population growth and food availability do affect health status and disease incidence.[2] And it is clear that deadly disease had a central function in Malthus's demographic models, as a major component of the misery that was both engendered by too rapid population growth and that helped to check population growth. It is true that Malthus's legacy with regard to issues of health is ambivalent: some will champion him as a pioneering analyst of the determinants of sustainable health, others will see Malthus as the originator of a set of arguments made in the name of natural necessity that challenge the very morality of much public health intervention.[3]

Yet the ambivalence of the legacy is probably not the main reason for neglect. Instead, it is the relation of population and political economy with the medical gaze that is problematic. It was problematic in Malthus's time and it still is. Where, that is, are we to locate the border between the problems of public medicine and the social and economic contexts in which those problems exist? Some will treat rates of population growth as a given, part of the conditions within which health problems must be solved. Others will see population control or some other socio-economic change as a part of the work of preventive medicine itself. Though such issues may be central in debates that take place in the interface where social medicine, development theory, and social philosophy meet, they are relatively invisible elsewhere in the dominions of medicine. The problem at the heart of Malthus scholarship, the one that continues to make him a figure of controversy, is an instance of this larger problem: are we to understand Malthus's project primarily as a descriptive or as a normative and prescriptive endeavor? Is he showing us what is or what should be? An exploration of issues of health and disease in the works of Malthus and his critics and commentators is a good way to illuminate central issues of this controversy.

'The sons and daughters of peasants will not be found such rosy cherubs in real life as they are described to be in romances,' wrote Malthus in the first edition of the *Essay on the Principle of Population*: even outside of periods of acute famine or of epidemic disease, the economic condition of the population could be read in the size and shape of the bodies of the populace.[4] While Malthus and his commentators and critics (these mostly defy disciplinary categorizations, but two, Thomas Jarrold and Charles Hall – discussed by Roy Porter elsewhere in this volume – were doctors) had a good deal to say about health and disease, their medical contemporaries had relatively little to say directly about Malthus's ideas. British medical men were, however, well acquainted with the effects of periodic scarcity on a population that lacked resources to cope with it, and with the high infant death rates of poverty. Much of what Malthus said about the 'positive check' of disease they would have agreed with – he got it from them, though usually indirectly.[5] On one level, the claim that fatal disease checked population was truistic. Many medical men generally agreed that a periodic disequilibrium between population and food was one of the scenarios that led to epidemic fever. The idea that squalor of any and every sort was more or less pathogenic was a commonplace and is reflected in the travel writings from which Malthus took so much of the material he would use in the later editions of the *Essay*. They were aware too, of the naturalizing discourse of Malthus and other political economists, in which such phenomena were seen to reflect the current state of a system of incentives and disincentives. But switching from analysis to policy, Malthus's ideas seemed anathema: the view of fatal disease as a natural solution to the population 'problem' could hardly accommodate the profession's public goal of healing and helping. Maybe the long-term health of all was threatened by the overabundance of some (which 'some' was key), but sounding that truth was no way to win patients.

To characterize their appraisals of Malthus's ideas and to distinguish them more clearly from those of political economists and other contemporary commentators on social policy, a tripartite classification of Malthusianism may help *(Figure 1)*. Most medical men who took an interest in population/health issues, if they accepted any of Malthus's findings at all, may be classified as *analytical or descriptive* Malthusians. They acknowledged such central elements of Malthus's theory as the concept of a redundant population. The tendency of population to grow more rapidly than food did adversely affect the health. Yet unlike most non medical commentators, who did feel an obligation to treat the issue as one of political economy, most were not *normative* or *prescriptive* Malthusians as well. They did not accept that the particular social and economic policies deduced by Malthus were the right ones, nor did they regard political economy as superceding the customary duties and sensibilities of medical professionals. Finally, one finds a few figures who are best labeled *ideological, vindictive,* or even *performative* Malthusians. These may be anti-Jacobins or the utilitarian Malthusians of dark Dickensian legend, who invoke

---

Figure 1

**Varieties of Malthusianism,
or, the population principle as axiom, tragedy, or polemic**

1. **Descriptive or Analytical Mathusianism:** The population principle is correct.

1a. Whether as an empirical inference or a deduction of economic law, it implies **no policy response** at all.

1b. At best it delineates **a policy problem,** but implies no particular solution. Many solutions exist; selection will require exogenous principles.

2. **Prescriptive Malthusianism:** The population principle is correct and the policies Malthus derives from it (marriage disincentives; abolition of poor law) are correct.

3. **Vindictive, Judgmental, Ideological Malthusianism:** the population principle and Malthus's derived policies are correct. They justify, generate, or reinforce contempt for the poor, the Irish, women, etc., and vindicate wealth and selfishness.

Malthus to justify class inequality or to discipline the dangerous classes.[6]

Our paper first outlines general areas of intersection of medicine and Malthus, mainly among English writers, and then turns to two case studies. The first examines the multiple readings of Malthus by Irish medical men interpreting the fever of 1817-19. The second focuses on the medical Malthusianism with which the Edinburgh medical professor William Pulteney Alison combated the economic Malthusianism of the Edinburgh divinity professor Thomas Chalmers in the Scottish poor law controversy of the early 1840s.

I

Why no noisy medical challenge to the Malthusians? Malthus seems to be suggesting that a state of unhealth is the normal lot for a large number of human beings, the best they can hope for, and the appropriate condition in terms of Providence. Some commentators noted, and pretty bluntly, that public medical intervention on a large scale was part of the problem. It exacerbated a situation that natural processes would resolve. The view was expressed by John Weyland, in the process of refuting it:

> If the world be already miserable because it has a continual tendency to repletion, all charity which encourages marriage among the lower orders in order to promote happiness and morality, which assists women in child-birth, which promotes vaccination and the cure of painful and distressing diseases, which helps in short any of the poor to rear their children in soundness of body, which bestows relief upon the old who have not saved a provision from their youthful earnings, which saves in any manner the life of one whose death would set his fellow creatures more at ease, is a criminal indulgence of individual feeling at the extent of the general welfare of mankind.[7]

(Ironically, Weyland appealed to a high and uncorrectable rate of urban mortality as the factor that would prevent disequilibrium between food and population.)

Surely a divided and beleaguered British medical profession would seize an opportunity to counter this depiction and vigorously to represent their art as on the side of life, health, and virtue.[8] And yet it did not. Two possibilities arise. One is that privately many medical men were vindictive Malthusians: the poor were too many and their high mortality no great loss. Edwin Chadwick believed this was the view of many of his poor-law-administrator colleagues, including some in the medical service, and ascribed to it the profession's disinterest in public health.[9] The view of medical students as jaded sensualists interested in the poor only as cadavers to cut goes along with this, but if there were many medical Malthusians they were quiet about it, while there were many who were openly advocates for the poor.[10]

More fruitful is the exploration of boundaries: that medical men saw, or came to see, population and poverty as beyond their competence, as appropriately a part of the emerging domain of political economy. Many would probably have rejected the presumption that underlies this paper, and would have held that economic causes of disease are no more a part of medical responsibility than are acts of God. Certainly most medical professionals did not follow radical critics of political economy to the view that the so-called population problem along with class-specific health problems, were due to class-injustice, capitalism, and bad property law. Instead, their consciousnesses unraised, poor law and charity medical staff patched up the slaughter of the industrial revolution.[11] Their focus, after all, was on the symptoms that 'presented' not populations and systems that presented them.

While such a dichotomous view may account for the response of the profession in general, it is important also to recognize that the boundaries were permeable and unfixed. Malthus himself crossed far into public medicine; medical men found themselves thinking about certain medical practices and institutions in terms of incentives and disincentives. On both sides, the picture is complex. At the conceptual level, deadly disease had a wide range of significations for Malthus and those who invoked his work. At the level of policy, the medicine-Malthus interface was very much issue-specific: foundling hospitals might be seen to have quite different implications from vaccination programs or public infirmaries.

Even in his antipopulation mode, Malthus was not uniformly antimedicine.[12] On many aspects of social intervention his views changed as he responded to critics. Population-slowing measures, like moral restraint or his proposal to withhold poor law rights from the not yet born, were to focus on those to come not those already aboard (or at the table, in his unfortunate and short-lived metaphor).[13] Medical interventions were to be assessed mainly in terms of incentives to irresponsible marriage: foundling hospitals were unacceptable; intervention in disease or accident was not – no one chose to become an accident victim; it did not reflect imprudence; had no bearing on marriage. Malthus stayed well back from the view that fatal disease was good (some tried to convict him of that);[14] in mature Malthusianism disease was mainly descriptive: it explained why things weren't more miserable.[15] Thus, what to some was Malthus's equivocation, to others his laudable rigor in assessing each intervention independently, did mitigate an inflammatory and polarized situation.[16]

Moreover, the Malthusian scenario of population constantly straining against resources could be read within very divergent narratives, and it is by no means the case that those who adopted a Malthusian analysis were opposed to a socializing medicine or that those who opposed Malthus were advocates of such a medicine. For neomalthusians, like George Drysdale and J. S. Mill, the narrative was liberation: Malthus's demonstration of a tendency toward overpopulation provided the empirical foundation for the practice of population control, which would eradicate domination and misery.[17] And population, as quantity or as growth rate, was not necessarily problematic. For Bishop Sumner and Southwood Smith the narrative was that of the discipline necessary for salvation.[18] They were the optimists; confronting the same situation, Sumner's brother bishop Philpotts saw mainly fallen man and woman and understood the population crisis also as a liberalism-squelching blessing. The struggle simply to survive damped social mobility and prevented escape from that godly institution, the barefoot and pregnant world of the rural Anglican parish.[19] Among Malthus's opponents, Michael Sadler shared Philpotts' view of the effects of overpopulation, but concluded that since that crisis was unjust it could not be providential.

By no means were all of those who, like Sadler, damned Malthus for endorsing misery and stealing from the poor their only remaining joy, the disinterested champions of universal human fulfillment.[20] Tory pronatalists envisioned happy parishes swarming with cannon fodder.[21] Some had no objection to misery, but only its supposed geometric growth, which conflicted with their notions of harmonious divine equilibrium: misery was fine so long as it knew its place. For Simon Gray, John Weyland, James Grahame and Michael Sadler, the status of towns as mortality sinks, particularly through high infant mortality, was providential and uncorrectable: it prevented a disequilibrium of subsistence and population in advanced civilized societies.[22]

We must also be careful not to attribute to orthodox medical men an insensitivity to the demand for antidotes to procreation. Familiar with families whose incomes barely sufficed for health, those with charity experience knew that the arrival of an additional mouth to feed threatened the equilibrium of survival.[23] Some wrote

sympathetically of parents' ambivalence toward a new baby or equally
to its death: small pox was said to be the poor man's friend. John
Roberton, surgeon to the Manchester Lying-in Hospital and author
of *Observations on the Mortality and Physical Management of Children*
(1827) reluctantly concluded that a relatively high level of infant
mortality was inescapable – one might well think that many children
were 'sent into the world ... for no purpose but to undergo a variety
of sufferings, and become the early victims of disease.' Like 'a
luxurious fruit tree; numerous blossoms are put forth, and afterward
abundant fruit: but of the blossoms, many are shed as ... they appear;
and of the fruit, much falls before it is full grown.' Much of this
mortality might be prevented, but even if all were done that might
be, Roberton estimated that the death rate before age ten would
remain at a level of 25–30%. Yet far from arguing that infant
mortality was a natural process with which medicine should not
meddle, he raised the point in denouncing 'a political
hardheartedness which would represent the most terrible diseases to
be *designed* as salutary checks to excessive population' and
complained that since Malthus 'many absurd, and some criminal,
notions have been promulgated on the subject of CHECKS to the
increase of mankind'.[24]

Nor were medical men so fixated on the clinical as to be oblivious
of the social causes of disease. Like Roberton, many saw poverty as a
chief predisposing cause, even if in the economists' view they were
naive in ignoring the deeper causes of poverty. But that very naivete
was, in a sense, profoundly radical: preoccupied with the immediate
and the material over the institutional or abstract, they concentrated
on pathogenic components of poverty – poor food, clothing, shelter,
heat, overcrowded housing. True it might be that the poor are with
us always, but surely a state could see that people had food, heat,
shelter, and contagion-inhibiting housing. That these factors caused
fatal disease was proof enough of their unacceptability. Focusing
narrowly, refusing the gambit of systems-talk, left no room to reject
the medical imperative. We doctors have no business with
economics; have what system you will, it must produce health – an
increasingly high standard of health, no less – and that is for we
doctors to determine. There are exceptions, doctors who did address
deeper causes. Charles Hall, M.D., devoted the first 30 pages of his
1805 anti-Malthusian work the *Effects of Civilization* to poverty's
pathogenic effects and the next three hundred to its causes, which, in
effect, he found to be capitalism.[25]

Whether or not medical men chose to acknowledge the social, they could not escape Malthus. The pervasive Malthusianism of the teens, twenties, and thirties intruded issue-by-issue into practice. We have mentioned foundling hospitals.[26] A striking feature of public health in the early Chadwickian era is the unwillingness to see infant mortality as a health problem in its own right (it was used as an indicator).[27] Most medical men met Malthus on the issue of poor-law medicine.[28] At issue was not so much the legitimacy of public care (Malthus was less vehement than some, who held that illness was culpable and could be avoided by making people bear its cost), but the view of the human subject. Briefly, where Malthus and most economists thought in terms of an integral self (in theory a male, in practice often a female) who responded rationally to necessity, medical men often imagined a fragile self, often gendered female, whose integrity could not be assumed. Where Malthus, Sumner, and Southwood Smith saw inequality as a providential means of generating industry, many poor law medical men recognized that indigence did not thus operate. Economic responsibility required physical and mental strength; poverty sapped strength; degradation led to further degradation: people did not respond to signals and prods; they simply had no hope and didn't care. Thus William Pulteney Alison, on whom more anon: in 'spring 1838, I saw three young women with natural children on the breast, ... out of work, in a miserable state of destitution, ... refused admission into the workhouses, ... scantily relieved by the other charities ... After some weeks of severe suffering, the children all died, certainly ... of cold and imperfect nourishment. If anyone supposes, that the effect of this sacrifice ... was to improve the morals of these women or their associates, ... he knows nothing of the effect of real destitution on human character and conduct.'[29]

The clash of outlooks was starkest in housing. Malthus had been convinced on his Scandinavia tour that in rural Norway cottage scarcity checked population: child-bearing was postponed to midlife because couples did not marry without a cottage. By limiting cottages, Britain might similarly control its population. If on almost every other population issue Malthus altered his view, here he did not waver. Conveniently his view undergirded the vision of some landowners' of the cottage- and hence rates-free estate where all one's workers lived in someone else's parish.[30] To a growing group of medico-sanitarian-moralists, however, cottage-destruction didn't work: It led not to prudence but to inappropriate agglomerations of human beings masquerading as family units. As foci of sexual knowledge and opportunity, crowded cottages promoted rather than retarded growth of a miserable population. And among the best accepted maxims of pathology was that concentrated human exhalations were the most common source of contagion and debilitation. As rising-expectations incentives began to displace misery disincentives at the end of Malthus's life, the hopes of both medicos and moralists came to rest on well-ventilated, single-family cottages.

II

In Ireland, more than anything, Malthus's influence was political, and it showed up in a political medicine that interpreted fever in Ireland in 1817-19. With the pervasiveness of Malthusianism in the late teens, the rapid growth of population in Ireland, and the centrality in Malthus's thought of epidemic disease as a positive check, it did not take a rocket scientist to see Ireland as a Malthusian exemplar, although Malthus himself was hesitant to make that assessment.[31] The Irish fever of 1817 to 1819 (a mix of typhus and relapsing fever) afflicted about 1.25 million people and killed about 65,000.[32] It was part of a widespread outbreak following a pan-European crop failure.[33] Irish medical men were pivotal in both national and local responses to the epidemic, investigating the epidemic, advising the government, and administering its public

---

Figure 2

**Summary of Views on the Social Causes and
Political Remedies of the Irish Fever, 1816–1819**

George Renny (1757–1848)
Poverty caused by Population is the cause ... No solution

John Cheyne (1777–1836)
Unemployment a cause ... incentives, paternalistic networks and expertise a solution

Francis Barker (d.1859)
Epidemic experience will drive expertise which will drive improvement

William Harty (1781–1854)
Contagion and transitory misery cause ... targeted interventions the solution

Whitley Stokes (1763–1845)
Contagion is the cause ... economic development the solution

---

response. Here we look at five Dublin-based medical men – George Renny (1757-1848), Francis Barker (*d.* 1859)[34], John Cheyne (1777-1836)[35], Whitley Stokes (1763-1845)[36], and William Harty (1781-1854).[37] Collectively, their views, which are summarized in Figure 2, make clear not only that medical men were thinking about the epidemic in terms of population-food issues, but also that an enormous range of descriptive and normative versions of the population problem had already become highly politicized.

George Renny was surgeon, and later physician to the Royal Hospital, Kilmainham from 1784, member of the Irish Army board from 1795, and Director General of [Army] Hospitals in 1817. Under the Irish Chief Secretary, Robert Peel, and under-secretary, William Gregory, he served on a three member committee allocating funds for fever assistance. Renny attributed fever to poverty and poverty to a very rapid population growth. The only medical man on the committee, he doubted the effectiveness of such funds in stopping fever. He wrote:

> It is ... evident ... that Fever will prevail ... while these predisposing causes continue to operate so extensively, and that we must look beyond medical ... exertions, for palliating or removing the present heavy affliction. .... Government ... may perhaps do something... but it is very difficult to find an effectual remedy for poverty, the causes of which are mainly ascribed to a rapidly increasing population, whilst the means of procuring productive ... employment for the multitude ... remains nearly stationary.[38]

Writing to Peel in May 1818, he defended the Fever Committee, but its actions were futile if Peel continued to limit its scope simply to stopping the fever.

> had We [*sic*] felt ourselves authorized to take a wider view of the Subject at the outset and comprehended within the Scope of relief the manifold privations of the lower orders, to which the cause and continuance of the exciting Epidemic are mainly to be ascribed, ... a Sum of money, would have been required ... the amount of which it would have been difficult to calculate, but which probably would have exceeded the most liberal policy.[39]

Renny even queried Peel's opinion on whether his authority would eventually sanction funds for convalescent Patients. Thus his Malthusianism was the reluctant acknowledgement of tragedy. Government money thrown at the epidemic could perhaps stop fever, but its predisposing cause, poverty induced by overpopulation, would still exist. 'Positive' checks of war and epidemics were tragic but unavoidable.

John Cheyne came to Dublin in 1809 with an Edinburgh M.D. During the fever epidemic he was physician to the Dublin House of Industry, co-author with Francis Barker of the main report on the fever epidemic, and the medical inspector for Leinster, appointed by Peel's successor, Charles Grant, in 1819. In 1820 he was appointed physician-general to the forces in Ireland, the highest Irish state medical post.

Cheyne did not specifically cite population as a cause of disease. He did see unemployment and economic distress as predisposing causes, and addressed these in terms of incentives, rather than legal, and costly public institutions. In his fever report of early 1819 Cheyne objected to establishment of more fever hospitals: they 'would afford the rich but too plausible an excuse for neglecting the indigent sick'.[40] And in terms similar to those of Malthus, he held that permanent fever hospitals would further weaken the Irish poor:

> By furnishing the poor with a ready asylum in their sickness, these institutions would have a tendency to make them even less provident than they are; ... they would still farther weaken that spirit of independence which ought to be encouraged in the poor of this country.[41]

Instead, fever hospitals should be provided only in times of distress. Boards of Health were not objectionable in principle, but in Leinster they had suffered from lack of 'persons of superior rank to protect and encourage them'.[42] Cheyne favored voluntary associations for poor relief. They were especially necessary in areas unable to maintain a Board of Health, and would augment charitable links between poor and rich without requiring government funds. To make these societies more efficient, a Board of Health in Dublin might supply information and assistance. Cheyne hoped this Dublin Board 'might also lay the foundation of general system of medical police'.[43]

Barker, also an Edinburgh M.D., promoter of the first Irish fever hospital and professor of chemistry at Trinity College Dublin, was physician to the Cork-Street Fever Hospital during the epidemic, and a member of the Health Subcommittee of the Association for the Suppression of Mendicity. He would serve as the Secretary to the permanent Board of Health in Ireland from 1820 until 1852.

In Barker's view the epidemic was a providential tragedy that would induce improvement in public health. In the October 1818 report of the Cork-Street hospital, he noted:

> Legislative interference has been obtained to aid the public in putting a stop to the present calamity, and preventing its future recurrence. Enlarged views have been acquired respecting ... fever, and an evil [of] ... formidable consequences has been at least comparatively mitigated. If ... the epidemic should gradually lead to an improvement in the habits, feelings, and condition of the whole community, that which appears ... a calamity, may ... prove the means of introducing health and happiness in the place of disease and misery.[44]

In 1819 Grant appointed Barker medical inspector in Munster. Like Cheyne, he believed that local associations for poor relief would allow the classes of society better to know each other. He too stressed paternalistic expertise:

> The distribution of publications ... from persons well informed on the state of the poor and the means of obviating sickness, and having sufficient authority, derived from knowledge and experience, to command attention, would also contribute to prevent or restrain the progress of fever.[45]

Other medical men, less optimistic, saw Malthusianism as an excuse for government inaction. William Harty, physician to the King's Hospital and to the prisons of Dublin, complained to Grant of the:

> pseudo-philanthropists, who can contemplate, not only without pain but with complacency, pestilence thinning the ranks of our 'superabundant' population; or to use the philosophic phraseology of our Malthite disciples, can with unalloyed satisfaction, behold fever 'doing its business'.[46]

By acknowledging poverty as a chief cause of fever and population as the chief cause of poverty, the Commons committee had unintentionally found itself in the position of seeing fever as the solution to fever:

> it would plainly follow, ... that [in order] to remove fever, which is the effect of poverty, we must check a rapidly encreasing population, [for which] fever is an efficient agent: therefore to remove fever, we must obviate poverty and to obviate poverty we should encourage fever.[47]

Harty focused instead on distinct and transitory components of poverty as fever causes: contagion and 'the miserable condition of the lower orders, arising from famine, want of employment, of cleanliness, and of fuel, and aggravated by despondency of mind.' These were remediable by a government not bound by Malthusian shackles.

Whitley Stokes,[48] a professor of medicine in the Royal College of Surgeons and a former United Irishman, likewise saw Malthusian analyses as blocking needed development in Ireland. He depicted the Malthusians as viewing hospitals, work-houses and quarantines as vain attempts 'to delay the thinning of the people, which is necessary to the happiness of mankind.'[49] He added that 'Mr. Malthus's system is ... particularly mischievous to Ireland' precisely because it seemed so resistant to the ordinary checks. 'Her population greatly increasing, is to his disciples an object of horror and aversion, the more from their feeding on those vile potatoes, and living in mud cabins – so circumstanced there is but a distant prospect of their perishing by famine – as earthquakes are rare in Ireland, war and pestilence are the only remedies from which timely relief can be expected. In the meantime, to everything that can contribute to keep up the overgrown population, they are coldly disposed.'[50] In September 1818 Stokes implored the government to reject Malthusian thinking and make health a priority:

> If Governments are anxious to prevent Idleness, Mendicity, Famine and outrage, [how] can they look on an evil that directly leads to Idleness, Mendicity, Famine and outrage? If they look for productive industry that shall replenish the coffers of their States do they hope it from the palsied hand of sickness? Can the dead labour? Can the dying labour? Can the unprotected orphan learn to labour for them on itself? If the health of the people is not a Government concern why was it made a subject of enquiry in Parliament? Why was an act passed last session on the subject of fever hospitals and boards of health? Why is a hospital endowed with funds for the purpose of preventing the extension of a venereal disease? If it is meritorious to restrain the extension of a disease which is communicated to the guilty, [is it] ... less so to restrain fever which effects the most virtuous and affectionate?[51]

The crucial medical question of how to deal with the epidemic became a politically charged issue to these medical men serving as either wanted or unwanted advisers to government officials. Was the fever epidemic just doing its business and acting as the Malthusian positive check to population? In an Irish context, Malthus and medicine intersected in the daily lives of medical men treating their fever patients.

III

Our second case is the medical Malthusianism of Dr. William Pulteney Alison, who in the late 1830s and early to mid 1840s led a campaign for a poor law for Scotland. In 1839 Alison was the leading member of the Edinburgh medical faculty. He held the chair in the Institutes of Medicine, and would soon succeed to that of the Practice of Medicine, which had been occupied by the great William Cullen, and was also physician to the New Town dispensary. If Alison is less known than Cullen as a medical systematist, he was enormously influential as a medical teacher, and was one of the last paragons of the application of the common sense philosophy to medicine. He exemplified a physician's career ideal: culture, learning, society, professional adroitness, commitment to medical charities, great compassion.

In response to the refusal of the General Assembly of the Church of Scotland to admit that its system of voluntary assessments for poor relief had failed to keep pace with migration and urbanization, Alison made the case for a guaranteed standard of relief and medical care in a pamphlet, *Observations on the Management of the Poor in Scotland, and its effects on the Health of Great Towns,* published in the spring of 1840. In the next few months, he supplemented this with more demographic treatments of the issues before the Statistical Society of London and the British Association, which met in Glasgow in September 1840.[52] His chief opponent was Rev. Thomas Chalmers, Bridgewater treatise author, leading evangelical, political economist, and architect of an approach to welfare provision that combined the harsh prod of nature with the scrutiny and exhortation of parish deacons. Chalmers worried that any recognition of a public right to relief would induce dependence and demoralization. He was a prescriptive Malthusian – but for the inspecting and exhorting deacons, his view of want as God's goad was that of Malthus and Sumner.[53] As Edinburgh divinity professor he was no longer a social administrator, yet the experiment in the Glasgow St. John's parish he had served in the 1820s remained the exemplar of the Scottish policy of attending jointly to the moral, spiritual, and, tangentially, the physical welfare of each soul. Malthus himself had endorsed the traditional Scottish approach, one which barely recognized any right to public relief. [54]

Alison, by contrast, was a descriptive Malthusian. He agreed that

128

a redundant population existed, though he understood redundancy less in terms of food than labor demand.[55] He saw a population/labor disequilibrium as the chief source of destitution, and, as a fever doctor, saw transient, destitute people, like those who came to Edinburgh from the highlands or Ireland as the chief source of contagious fever.

Alison largely rejected an economist's analysis based in hypothetical incentives to prudence. Instead, he based his case on pathological theory, a practitioner's ethic, and empirical study of the geography of destitution. He differed from Chalmers and Malthus in decoupling welfare from moral reformation. Moral reformation was fine, but a gap between the amount of work available and quantity of labor present to do it was not God's reminder to be virtuous, but only a pathological state of human society.

In appealing to an intensively biological concept of a human substrate, Alison commanded the field. Economists, after all, could not claim expertise in physiology or pathology, and the concept of significant externally caused human variability had little place in their analyses, either descriptively or normatively. Their human chooser was in effect a transcendent, disembodied, mind. If it breathed it was rational, and presumably chugged along evaluating options and allocating resources no matter what its stomach received or how congested its lungs became. If anything, the greater the exigencies, the sharper the rationality: the poor were more rational than the rich, who could afford to err (and good for all that they could, Malthus had proved).

But where the economist presumed universal competence, the doctor suspected widespread incompetence. Particularly in the Scottish nervous system-based pathology, the inviolate mental command-center was a fiction. Yes the mind was full of innate faculties, but they were many and their integration subject to derangement both by material forces – diet, exhaustion, heat, cold, air, contagia – and by immaterial: grief or anxiety for the future.[56] However uncomfortable they might have been with Owenism, medical theory pushed doctors toward the 'circumstances,' rather than the 'character' camp.[57]

Not only was the individual's constitution delicate, it was dangerously unbounded, capable of corrupting far beyond the individual soul. Even if one limited a conception of inescapable social relation to spreading diseases, Alison had a far grimmer view of the consequences of misery than did the Malthusians. Economic individualism presumed incentives and consequences to operate primarily on the individual as an economic unit, and saw its fate as mattering little to other units in parallel struggles (except insofar as its disappearance gave them easier access to scarce resources). But for Alison society was no collection of discrete units, but more like a mash of newly dyed cloths, each bleeding into the other.

One of the chief mechanisms of this miscible misery was continued fever, which was one of Alison's medical specialties. Like many other medical men he believed that it could generate spontaneously in debilitated people. It could then become contagious, even to the non-debilitated, even to the rich. (Indeed, the tone of some treatments of this pathology would warrant the appellation 'retributive fever'.) If economics operated on individuals, disease operated on populations. Humans were permeable; inequality did have social costs that economists failed to recognize: in disease, moral decay, and even, in the view of sanitarian statesmen like R. A. Slaney, in a revolution cost.[58]

The combined recognition of human fragility and of the hazard of incendiary disease led Alison to reject the usual demarcation of desert among the poor – the distinguishing of the few who might be excused from market participation due to incapacity from the many who must feel its full rigor. Physiology undermined this distinction, and astride the physiological analogy Alison crossed back into the land of the economists to argue that even in their terms, autonomy was fantasy.

Chalmers had admitted that those suffering from incurable disease or accident deserved medical charity on the grounds that those diseases signified acts of providence not individuals' choices. In fact, pure Providence was rare, replied Alison the experienced dispensary doctor: imprudence or intemperance were factors in very many cases, and a consistent consequences-based welfare system would have to deny care in them. But his main thrust was against Chalmers' concept of Providence itself. How, for example, to view that disabling 'visitation of Providence which the mere advance of years brings upon all.' To the argument that responsible agency entailed saving for one's old age, Alison objected that uncontrollable circumstances often prevented this. The same applied to destitution generally: 'Many ... are ... destitute, ... from causes over which they have had as little control as over the dispensations of Providence; ... failure of [an] industry in consequence of improvement in art, the glut of markets, commercial embarrassments from failure of banks ... or the general increase of population.' Where Chalmers was wanting to treat anyone not claiming charity as (economically) independent,

Alison was arguing that every laborer was (biologically) dependent: 'the moral and political dangers affecting his character... which are to be apprehended from the loss of his independence, *are already incurred.*'[59]

Most remarkable in Alison's discussion is the inclusion of population as an *exogenous* factor in the assessment of responsibility for one's condition. The thrust of Malthus' preventive check argument, after all, was that procreation was the seminal fount of *personal* responsibility. Overpopulation is no act of god, but their (our) doing in the most direct way. Surely if they (we) are made miserable by the overabundance of them (us), they (we) uniquely have the power to shut off the fount and remedy that misery. Alison's statement that we have 'as little control' over 'the general increase of population' as we do 'over the dispensations of Providence' does not mean that he thinks that babies pop out under cabbages; instead it reflects his view that population-food-labor imbalances are remediable public policy problems. He believed that there was food-growing potential sufficient for the existing population and that labor demand was more a matter of political institutions than of an independent process of capital accumulation. Like many of Malthus's critics, he touted wasteland reclamation schemes that promised work and food. In this way population took its place with general gluts or commercial failures as phenomena which, if not wholly avoidable, were certainly not the fault of the individual laborer. All these were events which societies needed to expect and for which they needed to plan.

Plainly, Alison saw the relation of individual to society quite differently than did Chalmers and Malthus, and this leads into our second point, the centrality of a practitioner's ethic in his argument and the associated conception of the individual that it brought with it. Despite its oft-mentioned individualism, political economy was not friendly to individuals, who it burdened with a huge load of historical situation. Malthus effectively made any individual in a population (or better a class) responsible for the condition of that population, despite the fact that redundant population was the outcome of multiple decisions in earlier generations. The approach was redolent with original sin; sins (quite literally of fathers, presumably the choosers) fall on sons; there need be no apology if anyone's range of choice was curtailed by irresponsible decisions of ancestors or competitors. But if a continual flux in which no one's experience merited the privilege of subjectivity was perhaps essential to an economist's analysis, it was not to a doctor's.

Alison's was, one is tempted to say, a more consistent concept of responsibility. To the degree that they were functional and free, individuals bore responsibility for their own actions. But they were not responsible for the historical situation into which they had been deposited. Where Chalmers saw relief to a child as problematic because it undermined the incentives that were supposed to keep its father working to support it, Alison objected to thus holding the child's health hostage. The same argument applied to wives, elderly dependents, and ultimately, even to adult males. It reflects the climate of dispensary practice: the symptoms that present are episodes in individual bodies. One does not treat economic units, much less economic systems; that fathers are profligate doesn't alter the medical condition of children.[60] The symptoms may implicate family or place, or at some greater distance political acts, but the person experiencing the symptoms is hardly in a position to do anything about those causes, and hence blame- or responsibility-talk is futile. Surely, if people had the capacity to make choices that would not end them up in dispensaries, they would have made them. It was, wrote Alison, 'no answer to ... statements, shewing a great redundancy of population in Scotland, to observe that many of these persons are ... profligate ..., and that their want of employment is to be ascribed to that cause. In many cases this is true, and in many others it is not true; but what concerns us at present is not the characters of the individuals, but the fact of their number being in excess.'[61]

While Alison acknowledged a duty of charity unqualified by the casuistry of desert, there was more than do-gooderism and epidemiology in his challenge to orthodox Malthusianism.[62] He held that destitution did not in fact function as a preventive check. Hungry adults were supposed to realize that they and any children they had would be hungrier the more of them they had, and restrain themselves. But as even Malthus knew, people with little to lose and little hope of gaining anything, and exhausted by mere survival, had neither rationale nor strength to practice bourgeois disciplines. Ireland and Scotland, without legal provision for the poor, showed much higher fertility rates than England, which had it; within Ireland and Scotland rates were highest in the most desperate populations.[63] Many economists were coming to agree that the incentive of 'artificial wants and habits of comfort' was more powerful as an incentive than the prospect of scarcity, and that it was thus good policy to make upward mobility possible through cheap goods, housing and sanitation, as well as through religion and education. Alison's argument paralleled theirs, but here too it was grounded in a more complex psychology.[64] Upward mobility required human dignity, which was a physiological state. The mental machine of the free person, which aspired and acted to achieve aspirations required a quantum of well-being. A reliable physiological safety net was a prerequisite for responsible reproduction.

IV

These cases suggest the inescapability of Malthusian issues for medical men. On the one hand the matter of deadly disease, some of it engendered by deprivation, had central demographic importance as a check to population; on the other hand any discussion of effective public medicine took place in terms set out by Malthus. The substantial presence of Malthus's ideas in public life demanded that those who practiced various forms of public health medicine reckon with the issues of the systemic causes of disease and of the systemic implications of their work. But even among those who endorsed aspects of it, Malthus's work was read in widely differing ways and taken to imply many different things, while those who cast themselves as critics of Malthus often accepted a great deal of his demonstrations, and in some cases placed even greater stress on the inexorable check of deadly disease. Accordingly, it is unhelpful to characterize the discussion in terms of pro- and anti-Malthus. It is however useful to recognize a tension between a predominantly medical framework for assessing issues of health and welfare and one which was predominantly economic. For the most part, the medical framework has been subordinated to the economic. That subordination is embodied in the identities of professions and public institutions as well as more broadly shared expectations and conventions of assessment: after all, we all know what political economy is; by comparison, a political or social medicine is nebulous and barely visible.[65] While the evolution of that tension during the rest of the nineteenth and the twentieth century is a complex story, the origins of that subordination lie in the period under study, we suggest, where Malthus met the doctors.

Notes

1   The omission is the more remarkable given the blossoming of
      scholarship on the interrelations of theology and political economy.
      See Boyd Hilton, *The Age of Atonement: The Influence of
      Evangelicalism on Social and Economic Thought, 1785-1865* (Oxford:
      Clarendon, 1988); A. M. C. Waterman, 'Malthus as a Theologian:
      the *First Essay* and the Relation between Political Economy and

Christian Theology' in J. Dupâquier, A. Fauve-Chamoux, and E. Grebenik (eds), *Malthus Past and Present* (London: Academic Press, 1983), 195–209; *idem, Revolution, Economics, and Religion: Christian Political Economy, 1798-1833* (Cambridge: Cambridge University Press, 1991); J. M. Pullen, 'Malthus' Theological Ideas and the Influence on his Principle of Population' *History of Political Economy* 13 (1981): 39–54; M. B. Harvey-Phillips, 'Malthus' Theodicy: the Intellectual Background of his Contributions to Political Economy' *History of Political Economy* 16 (1984): 591–608; Donald Winch, *Riches and Poverty: An Intellectual History of Political Economy in Britain, 1750-1834* (Cambridge: Cambridge University Press, 1996). It is quite true that historical demographers address such issues, and hence it is all the more interesting that scholarship on Malthus himself largely does not.

2   For a recent review see Helen Epstein, 'Life and Death on the Social Ladder', *New York Review of Books,* 16 July 1998, 26–9. See also Simon Szreter, 'Economic Growth, Disruption, Deprivation, Disease and Death: on the importance of the politics of public health for development', *Population and Development Review* 23 (1997), 693–728.

3   Anthony McMichael, *Planetary Overload : Global Environmental Change and the Health of the Human Species* (Cambridge: Cambridge University Press, 1993). These issues are implicated in the controversy about how far health will improve through designated health policies as distinct from economic development.

4   T. R. Malthus, *An Essay on the Principle of Population and A Summary View of the Principle of Population,* edited with an introduction by Anthony Flew (Harmondsworth, U.K.: Pelican, 1970), 93–4. Malthus goes on to note that nineteen year olds are mistaken for fifteen year olds, and that the plough boys, despite their exercise, do not have thick calves, both of which he attributes to 'lack of proper or of sufficient nourishment'.

5   In the first essay Malthus is somewhat tentative about the pathological impact of deprivation, and cites Süssmilch as his principal source (*An Essay on the Principle of Population,* 109). In later editions that tentativeness is largely gone. Cf fn 14.

6   On anti-Jacobinism and political economy see Waterman, *Revolution, Economics,* 7, 56.

7   John Weyland, *The Principles of Population and Production as they are affected by the Progress of Society with a view to moral and political consequences* (1816 rpt; New York: Kelley, 1969), 334.

8   On the state of the profession see especially Anne Digby, *Making a*

Malthus and the Doctors

Medical Living: Doctors and Patients in the English Market for Medicine, 1720-1911 (Cambridge: Cambridge University Press, 1994); I. Loudon, *Medical Care and the General Practitioner* (Oxford: Clarendon Press, 1986).

9   R. A. Lewis, *Edwin Chadwick and the Public Health Movement, 1832-1854* (London: Longmans, Green, 1952), 64.

10 Ruth Richardson, *Death, Dissection, and the Destitute* (London: Pelican, 1989).

11 Christopher Hamlin, *Public Health and Social Justice in the Age of Chadwick: Britain 1800-1854* (Cambridge: Cambridge University Press, 1998), chapters 1–2; Loudon, *Medical Care and the General Practitioner,* 130–1.

12 Whether Malthus saw rapid population growth, or the tendency toward population growth as truly problematic (in the sense of requiring to be solved) will depend on which texts one cites and is likely always to be for argument. But see Donald Winch, 'Robert Malthus: Christian Moral Scientist, Arch-Demonizer or Implicit Secular Utilitarian' *Utilitas* 5 (1993), 239–52; Gunnar Heinsohn and Otto Steiger, 'The Rationale Underlying Malthus's Theory of Population', in J. Dupâquier, A. Fauve-Chamoux, and E. Grebenik (eds), *Malthus Past and Present,* (London: Academic Press, 1983), 223–32.

13 For changing views on poor laws see Patricia James, *Population Malthus: His Life and Times* (London: Routledge and Kegan Paul, 1979), 374, 450–1.

14 T.R. Malthus, *An Essay on the Principle of Population; or A view of its past and present Effects on Human Happiness; With an Inquiry into our Prospects respecting the future Removal or Mitigation of the Evils which it Occasions, The version published in 1803, with the variora of 1806, 1807, 1817, and 1826,* 2 vols, II, 'appendix, 1817', Patricia James (ed.), (Cambridge: Cambridge University Press/Royal Economic Society, 1989), 233–4.

15 Malthus, *Essay on the Principle of Population* (James edition), I, 72, 93, 288–301. Cf II, 89.

16 William Peterson goes so far as to suggest that Malthus's legacy has been distorted by the elevation of 'emprical or logical points' into 'disputes about fundamental political or moral issues' (Peterson, *Malthus* [Cambridge MA: Harvard University Press, 1979], 80).

17 Francis Place, *Illustrations and Proofs of the Principle of Population, with critical and textual notes by Norman E Himes* (London: George Allen and Unwin, 1930); Place, 'documents on birth control, 1822', Francis Place Collection, British Library, sect 68, mf #50; [George

Drysdale], 'Statement of the Social Problem: The Law of Population
and its Effects', *The Political Economist; and Jouranl of Social Science*
1, nos. 1, 2 (1856), 3–16.

18 John Bird Sumner, *A Treatise on the Records of the Creation, and on
the Moral Attributes of the Creator; with particular reference to the
Jewish History, and to the Consistency of the Principle of Population
with the Wisdom and Goodness of the Deity,* 2 vols, 2nd edition
(London: Hatchard, 1818), II, ch. 3–5; Thomas Southwood Smith,
*Illustrations of Divine Government; First American from the last
London edition* (Boston: B. Mussey, 1831), 109–24.

19 R. A. Soloway, *Prelates and People: Ecclesiastical Social Thought in
England 1783-1852* (London: Routledge and Kegan Paul, 1969),
143–4; cf. 172–80.

20 Michael Sadler, *A Refutation; of an Article in the Edinburgh Review,
(no. CII.), entitled 'Sadler's Law of Population, and Disproof of Human
Superfecundity'* (London: John Murray, 1830), 9.

21 James Grahame, *An Inquiry into the Principle of Population, with a
New Introduction by Chuhei Sugiyama and Andrew Pyle* (1816; rpt.
London: Routledge/Thoemmes Press, 1994), 96–7, 208.

22 Simon Gray, *The Happiness of States; or, an Inquiry concerning
Population, the Modes of Subsisting and Employing It, and the Effects of
All on Human Happiness* (London: Hatchard, 1815), 351–3; John
Weyland, *The Principles of Population and Production,* 64, 110,
418–23; James Grahame, *An Inquiry into the Principle of Population,*
167; Michael Sadler, *The Law of Population, being a Treatise in Six
Books, in Disproof of the Superfecundity of Human Beings, and
Developing the Real Principle of their Increase,* 2 vols (London: John
Murray, 1830), I, 307–9; II, 76–7.

23 John Ferriar, 'Of the Prevention of Fevers in Great Towns', *Medical
Histories and Reflections,* 1st American edition, 4 vols in 1
(Philadelphia: Dobson, 1816), II, 235–9.

24 John Roberton, *Observations on the Mortality and Physical Mangement
of Children* (London: Longman, Rees, Orme, Brown, 1827), 3–10.

25 Charles Hall, *The Effects of Civilization on the People In European
States; with Observations on the Principal Conclusion in Mr. Malthus's
Essay on Population* (New York: Augustus M. Kelley, 1965).

26 On the effect of Malthusian ideas on foundling hospitals, see Ruth
McClure, *Coram's Children: The London Foundling Hospital in the
Eighteenth Century* (New Haven: Yale University Press, 1981),
252–3.

27 Hamlin, *Public Health and Social Justice in the Age of Chadwick,* 231;
Michael Sadler, *The Law of Population,* 2 vols (London: John

Murray, 1830), II, 159.

28 See Ruth Hodgkinson, *The Origins of the National Health Service:*
    The Medical Services of the New Poor Law, 1834-1871 (London:
    Wellcome Historical Medical Library, 1967).

29 William Pulteney Alison, *Observations on the Management of the Poor*
    in Scotland, and its Effects on the Health of Great Towns, 2nd edition
    (Edinburgh: Blackwood, 1840), 80 fn.

30 Harold Boner, *Hungry Generations: the Nineteenth-Century Case*
    against Malthusianism (New York: King's Crown Press, 1955), 54,
    58–9; Patricia James, *Population Malthus: His Life and Times*
    (London: Routledge and Kegan Paul, 1979), 73; J. R. Poynter,
    Society and Pauperism: English Ideas on Poor Relief, 1795-1834
    (London: Routledge and Kegan Paul, 1969), 219; G. Talbot Griffith,
    Population Problems in the Age of Malthus, 2nd edition (New York:
    Augustus M. Kelley, 1967), 80; Raymond Cowherd, *Political*
    Economists and the English Poor Laws: A Historical Study of the
    Influence of Classical Economics on the Formation of Social Welfare
    Policy (Athens, OH: Ohio University Press, 1977), 179, 198–9; K.
    Smith, *The Malthusian Controversy,* 70.

31 Malthus to Ricardo, July 1817, in Piero Sraffa (ed.), *The Works and*
    Correspondence of David Ricardo, Vol. VII, (Cambridge: Cambridge
    University Press, 1952), 175. Malthus himself visited Ireland on a
    family vacation in 1817 and wrote to his friend, Ricardo, 'Through
    most of this country, great marks of improvement were observable,
    though its progress had received a severe check during the last two
    years, the effect of which was peculiarly to aggravate the predominant
    evil of Ireland, namely a population greatly in excess above the
    demand for labour, though in general not much in excess above the
    means of subsistence on account of the rapidity with which the
    potatoes have increased under a system of cultivating them on very
    small properties rather with a view to support than sale.' See also
    Peterson, *Malthus,* 109. As Winch notes, Malthus himself, in an
    anonymous review, puzzled over the fact that more attention was not
    given to Ireland in the works of Malthus (Winch, *Riches and Poverty,*
    342). Malthus's writings on Ireland are reprinted in B. Semmel (ed.),
    Occasional Papers of T.R. Malthus (New York: Burt Franklin, 1963).

32 Francis Barker and John Cheyne, *An Account of the Rise, Progress, and*
    Decline of the Fever lately Epidemical in Ireland together with
    Communications from Physicians in the Provinces and Various Official
    Documents 2 vols (London: Baldwin, Cradock, and Joy, 1821), I, 63
    and 145; and Charles Murchison, *A Treatise on the Continued Fevers*
    of Great Britain (London: Parker, Son, and Bourn, 1862).

33 John Post, *The Last Great Subsistence Crisis in the Western World* (Baltimore, MD: Johns Hopkins University Press, 1977), 48. In this work, Post describes how severe weather in 1816 and 1817 devastated European agricultural output.

34 *Dictionary of National Biography*, vol. 1, 1119.

35 *Dictionary of National Biography*, vol. 4, 220.

36 *Dictionary of National Biography*, vol. 18, 1288.

37 *Dictionary of National Biography*, vol. 9, 77.

38 Select Committee Report, 'On Contagious Fever in Ireland', P.P. 1818 (825) Vol. VII.

39 *Peel Papers*, Vol. XCVII, BL Add MS 20277, May 8, 1818, Renny to Peel.

40 Appendix to the First Report from the Select Committee Report, 'Ireland: Disease, State of, and Condition of the Labouring Poor', 1819 (314), Vol. VIII, 81.

41 *Ibid.*, 81.

42 *Ibid.*, 82.

43 *Ibid.*

44 Francis Barker, M.D., *Medical Report of the Fever Hospital, Cork-Street, Dublin; Containing an Account of the Present Epidemic*, October 1, 1818, 599–600.

45 'Appendix to the First Report from the Select Committee Report on the State of Disease, Etc. in Ireland, 1819', 24.

46 William Harty, *An Historic Sketch of the Causes, Progress, Extent, and Mortality of the Contagious Fever Epidemic in Ireland During the Years 1817, 1818, and 1819* (Dublin: Hodges and M'Arthur, 1820), vi–viii.

47 Harty, *An Historic Sketch*, vi–viii.

48 Father of Dr. William Stokes of later medical fame.

49 Whitley Stokes, M.D., *Observations on the Population and Resources of Ireland* (Dublin: Joshua Porter, 1821), 10.

50 *Ibid.*

51 National Archives of Ireland, *Official Papers I*, OP 474/62.

52 W. P. Alison, 'Illustrations of the Practical Operation of the Scottish System of Management of the Poor', *Quarterly Journal, Statistical Society of London* 3 (1840), 211–57, esp. 246, 254, 217. See also Alison, *Reply to the Pamphlet entitled 'Proposed Alteration of the Scottish Poor Law Considered and commented on, by David Monypenny, esq. of Pitmilly'* (Edinburgh: Blackwood, 1840); *idem*, *Reply to Dr Chalmers' Objections to an Improvement of the Legal Provision for the Poor in Scotland* (Edinburgh: Blackwood, 1841). For a fuller discussion of the controversy and its place in the formulation

of public health policies see Hamlin, *Public Health and Social Justice*,
Chapter 4; Olive Checkland, 'Chalmers and William Pulteney
Alison: A Conflict of Views on Scottish Social Policy', in A.C.
Cheyne (ed.), *The Practical and the Pious: Essays on Thomas
Chalmers*, (Edinburgh: St. Andrew Press, 1986), 130–40.

53 Malthus found Chalmers to be far too dogmatic a representative of
his ideas (Winch, *Riches and Poverty*, 381–5).

54 Malthus, *An Essay on the Principle of Population*, (James edition),
'Appendix, 1817', 236.

55 W. P. Alison, 'Further Illustrations of the Practical Operation of the
Scotch System of Management of the Poor', *Quarterly Journal,
Statistical Society of London* 4 (1841), 288–319. Statistical study
should be concerned with 'the *extension of the population*, as
proportioned to the demand for labour, on which, of course, the
probability of the recurrence or permanence of the evils of
destitution depends' (290). Like most political economists, Alison
opposed aid in wages as interfering with labor demand (291).

56 On the links between Edinburgh medicine and philosophy see
Anand Chitnis, *The Scottish Enlightenment and Early Victorian
English Society* (London: Croom Helm, 1986), 13; Christopher
Lawrence, *Medicine as Culture: Edinburgh and the Scottish
Enlightenment* (PhD thesis, London: University of London, 1984).

57 A striking example of this difference in outlook is the construal of
the common phrase 'necessaries of life' in medical and economic
contexts. In the economic literature the 'necessaries' are those class-
specific elements of a standard of living whose maintenance governs
economic decision making – i.e. a carriage is necessary for a doctor,
who cannot marry if this entails giving it up. In the medical
literature the necessaries are the physical elements of subsistence
whose inadequate provision sustains only a less than adequate
condition of life (Cf. Hamlin, *Public Health and Social Justice*,
Nassau Senior, *Two Lectures on Population*, chap. 1 [London: John
Murray, 1831], 3–5).

58 Hamlin, *Public Health and Social Justice*, 246–8.

59 Alison, 'Illustrations', 246.

60 *Ibid.*, 255.

61 *Ibid.*, 217.

62 *Ibid.*, 253.

63 *Ibid.*, 255; Cf. 'Further Illustrations', 293: 'the general redundancy
of the population, [was] greatest in districts where the existing Poor
Laws are not enforced, and where the legal relief given is admitted to
be illusory; and, in connection with this the extension of epidemic

disease'.

64 Alison, *Illustrations*, 245.
65 The fate of concepts of social medicine has been well studied in the works of Dorothy Porter, for example, *Health, Civilization, and the State* (London: Routledge, 1999).

7

Malthusian Mutations:

The changing politics and moral meanings of birth control in Britain

Lesley A. Hall

In Britain, the term 'Malthusian' has persistently been employed not merely to describe the theories advanced by the Reverend Thomas Robert Malthus but also the arguments made on the basis of those theories for the employment of prudential checks to conception – the perhaps more accurate term 'neo-malthusianism' has rather seldom been used in the British context. This revisionist usage of the term 'Malthusian' has itself been subject to considerable slippage, being employed over a lengthy span of the later nineteenth and earlier twentieth centuries very generally as a euphemism for the practice of artificial birth control, without any particular reference to political economy justifications for the benefits of small families: readers of Aldous Huxley's 1932 dystopia *Brave New World* will recall the 'Malthusian belts' of contraceptives worn by the female characters. It can also be argued that arguments for the employment of birth control which were substantially, if not explicitly, Malthusian, have continued to be advanced well into the twentieth century and that contraception has been used by individual couples for essentially, though not necessarily articulately, Malthusian reasons. This paper thus considers 'malthusianism' as a recurrent element in the history of birth control in Britain rather than constituting a particular phase which can be distinguished from others during which contraception was conceptualised as 'eugenics', 'birth control', 'family planning', and so on. An enduring deployment of 'malthusianism' on what must be considered feminist grounds will also be explored, since from its earliest days British malthusian literature envisaged women's bodies as a resource to be protected from depletion by the use of prudential checks to conception (though sometimes also as a resource to be liberated for sexual indulgence without procreation).

Eighteenth-century prescriptive writings on marriage (as opposed to the oral and literary culture of male libertinage, or indeed female oral subcultures) had laid more emphasis on fecundity than restricting births, although this is not necessarily any guide to actual practice.[1] Folk knowledge of abortifacients had existed for centuries and preparations to bring about miscarriage figure in surviving manuscript receipt books. Apart from this, evidence for the practice of abortion is scanty, though presumably there was a female subculture within which information was passed on orally. Prior to 1803 procuring an abortion before quickening occurred had not been considered a crime and the frequency of such acts is therefore impossible to calculate. It only became a statutory offence in that year and abortion was increasingly criminalized during the nineteenth century (though the aborting women herself was seldom penalized, as opposed to third-party abortionists), although well into the twentieth century women still believed that attempts to 'bring on the period' early in pregnancy were permissible.[2]

The manufacture of condoms in Britain, and therefore, it may be presumed, their use, can be traced back to the seventeenth century from archaeological evidence unearthed at Dudley Castle in the Midlands. The animal gut condoms found during excavations there can be dated with considerable accuracy as having been made and used sometime prior to 1647. Literary references from the early eighteenth century tend to indicate, however, that the primary purpose of these appliances was the prevention of venereal disease, and condoms were thus strongly associated with a raffish libertine subculture.[3] There was a flourishing trade in handmade sheaths in London by the 1750s. We do not know if either condoms, abortifacients, or the range of other expedients described by Angus McLaren in *Reproductive Rituals*[4] were being used as means for the 'prudential restraint' of family size and whether there was an unnamed proto-Malthusianism already occurring, as McLaren has argued in *Sexuality and Social Order* to have been the case in eighteenth-century France,[5] or whether they were being employed to elude particularly inconvenient pregnancies in or outside marriage. It has never been a legal offence as such under British law to practice birth prevention or to purvey devices for that purpose, although the trade in appliances and any published discussion of the subject were severely circumscribed by laws relating more generally to obscenity.

In 1798 Malthus demonstrated in his *Essay on the Principles of Population* that population will always tend to multiply faster than the means of subsistence. Delayed marriage, or moral restraint, were the only means he advocated to control population, lumping artificial methods under the general heading of 'vice'. It was not long, however, before other thinkers, in particular those influenced by the Utilitarianism of Jeremy Bentham, suggested that human ingenuity might modify the iron laws advanced by Malthus. In 1819 James Mill (father of John Stuart Mill) implied in an article in the *Encyclopaedia Britannica* that there were means by which the relentless growth of population might be checked, though without giving details.[6]

In 1822 radical working class reformer Francis Place published *Illustrations and Proofs of the Principle of Population*, putting the case for the employment of 'precautionary means' by married persons, although rather than being a practical guide, it advanced a social theory for the employment of contraception.[7] In the next year Place produced his 'diabolical handbills' intended to disseminate the practical knowledge of contraception, 'To the Married of Both Sexes' recommending the female vaginal sponge to prevent large families leading to poverty. John Stuart Mill, then aged 17, was imprisoned for distributing birth control leaflets, possibly these publications by Place.[8] In 1826 Richard Carlile, freethinker and associate of Place, published *Every Woman's Book; or, What is Love* describing the sponge, condom and other means of preventing conception. A recent study of Carlile, however, argues that he was a rather late convert to malthusianism, with considerable ambivalence towards it, and that for him it formed one more supporting argument for his agenda of liberating female sexuality for the wider benefit of society.[9] His doctrines were further disseminated in the journal *The Republican* which he edited and the *Newgate Monthly Magazine* produced by his assistants while he was in prison for blasphemy.[10]

Both Place and Carlile had their roots in the 'radical underworld' of Regency Britain, in which political radicalism was allied to unconventional, even libertine, sexual morality, and a knowledge of political economy could be combined with practical expedients associated with prostitution and libertinage. This alliance was already disintegrating by the time they published these works recommending the prevention of conception. Their doctrines encountered opposition even in radical, freethinking circles as political radicalism was becoming increasingly allied with respectability, while politically hard-hitting libertine satire was mutating into cynically commercial pornography lacking subversive intent.[11] However, birth control was not universally anathematized amongst early nineteenth-century radicals and socialists. Robert Owen repudiated strictly Malthusian prophecies of over-population, arguing that rational production and distribution of resources would obviate scarcity, but seems to have made contraceptives available in his New Lanark factory. His son, Robert Dale Owen, made an explicit case for birth control in *Moral Physiology*, 1830. As with Carlile, political economy was an argument subsidiary to liberating sexual pleasure from procreation and putting the right to control their own fertility in women's hands.[12]

Arguments that smaller families would be beneficial to women's health and their functioning as mothers were thus already being advanced by these early neo-malthusian propagandists alongside the case for their beneficial impact on a family's economic status. Both Place and Carlile recommended methods – predominantly the sponge – which could be used by the woman. This foreshadowing of her own agenda seems to have been written out of the history of contraception by the well-known early twentieth-century birth control campaigner, Marie Stopes, in order to promote her claim to be advancing a whole new woman-centred discourse of contraception in the context of sexual pleasure. However, it would appear that early nineteenth century women in radical circles were inclined to be somewhat ambivalent about birth control, especially when this was presented in a context of free love, even when they did envisage happier and more equal relationships between the sexes eventually coming to pass.[13] While the freethinker, feminist and Owenite socialist Emma Martin (1821-1851), Barbara Taylor suggests, probably gave lectures and advice on contraception from her home in Covent Garden, this seems to have been unusual if not unique.[14] Janet Farrell Brodie suggests that the description of women's bodily functions by female health lecturers in antebellum America was considered quite shocking enough without any explicit discussion of birth control.[15]

In 1854 George Drysdale published *Physical, Sexual and Natural Religion* anonymously as 'by a Student of Medicine'. It put a detailed case for contraception but gave minimal practical information and was explicitly feminist, arguing that 'the development of woman [has] been crippled and impeded by man's interference', and making a strong case for women studying medicine, a cause to which Drysdale gave practical assistance.[16] While, as Miriam Benn has pointed out in her collective biography of the Drysdale family, *Predicaments of Love*, Drysdale had been brought up among the intellectual elite of Edinburgh, there is little evidence that he had had any prior contact with the radical freethought circles through which the malthusian doctrines of an earlier generation had been disseminated.[17]

His book was published by Edward Truelove, a freethought

publisher, but Truelove does not seem to have been Drysdale's first choice: he was, rather, the only publisher prepared to take the risk of issuing *Physical, Sexual, and Natural Religion*. As *Elements of Social Science* the book was repeatedly republished well into the twentieth century, kept in print at a low price through Drysdale's own subsidy.[18] There was little notice taken of the volume beyond the organs of freethought and secularist circles with which Truelove was associated and of which Drysdale became a part: and even there it was not universally approved. Advocacy of preventive checks was capable of dividing the secularist movement and the accusation of promoting immorality was deployed as a weapon in internal battles.[19]

An early Malthusian League to promote the doctrines of prudential restraint was set up during the 1860s by Charles Bradlaugh, freethinker, radical, and journalist, but little is known about it. Bradlaugh also published articles on the subject in his journal *National Reformer*, and his praise in its columns for *Physicial, Sexual, and Natural Religion* led to his co-editor's resignation and a schism in the secularist movement.[20] Birth control, therefore, was advocated by the radical fringe of a radical fringe. The most tentative attempts to discuss family limitation met furious objection from the press and public opinion. Viscount Amberley (the father of Bertrand Russell) addressed the London Dialectical Society in 1868 suggesting that small families were desirable and means of limitation should be discussed (according to Russell's autobiography, Amberley himself practised contraception within his marriage, though the family claimed that this had made him epileptic[21]). As a result he was subjected to furious attacks by both the medical and lay press and lost a Parliamentary election amid the display of obscene cartoons 'representing his lordship selling certain quack mixtures to prevent large families' and scenes of riot.[22]

In 1877 Charles Bradlaugh and his colleague Annie Besant produced a cheap edition, with notes by Drysdale, of the American Charles Knowlton's birth control tract *Fruits of Philosophy*, as a test case of the law. They were tried for publishing 'a dirty, filthy book', although the verdict which was finally achieved was ambiguous (along the lines that the book was obscene but their intentions were not). Besant herself wrote and published a sixpenny pamphlet, *The Law of Population*, giving the case for contraception and providing information about the methods currently available, which was not prosecuted.[23] However, a number of other individuals – including Edward Truelove, prosecuted for publishing Robert Dale Owen's *Moral Physiology* – who published or distributed malthusian literature did come into conflict with the law, the operations of which were somewhat haphazard.[24]

In the same year as the Bradlaugh-Besant trial, 1877, a new Malthusian League was set up with C. R. Drysdale (George Drysdale's brother) as President and Annie Besant as secretary. It produced a regular monthly journal from 1879. Until 1914 it concentrated its endeavours on putting the general case for the benefits of family limitation, rather than giving specific advice, although recommended reading on this subject appeared in *The Malthusian*.[25] The League's arguments consciously appealed to archetypal 'Victorian values' of prudence, foresight and self-help. However, it is quite clear that the prevalent view at that time was that sex was not an area in which prudence and foresight were appropriate – except from the point of view of avoiding temptation and maintaining continence, i.e., not doing it.

The preconceptions which ruled large swathes of Victorian society, even those parts of it which would have considered themselves enlightened and forward looking, are revealed by the experience of Alice Vickery, Katherine Mitchell and Mrs Julia Mitchell Swaagman of the Malthusian League, who were among the earliest women to apply to the London School of Medicine for Women, in 1877. Vickery had indeed been a defence witness at the Bradlaugh-Besant trial and was not merely a member of the Malthusian League but one of its Vice-Presidents. The Council of the School, composed of individuals prepared to devote themselves to the controversial cause of women's medical education, had considerable anxieties that this connection might have undesirable repercussions on the struggle for medical degrees for women. Vickery, Mitchell and Swaagman were thus constrained to guarantee that their names would not be publicly linked with the Malthusian League during their association with the School.[26]

The teachings of the Malthusians were violently attacked on a combination of medical and moral grounds by C. H. F. Routh, in a paper given to the Obstetrical section of the British Medical Association in 1878: *On the Moral and Physical Evils likely to follow if practices intended to act as Checks to Population be not strongly discouraged and condemned*.[27] This exemplified the recurrent pattern whereby the British medical profession tried extremely hard to ignore malthusianism (and indeed various other manifestations of sexuality which could not be subsumed to procreative matrimony), but burst forth in condemnatory diatribes when provoked by events in the lay world such as the Amberley affair and the Bradlaugh-Besant trial.

There cannot be said to have been any sustained medical debate on the subject.[28]

In 1886 a radical doctor in Leeds, Yorkshire, Henry Arthur Allbutt, published *The Wife's Handbook*, a cheap manual for women on the preservation of health which included a brief chapter on the prevention of conception when medically advisable, and thus formed part of a continuing case for birth control being made on grounds of maternal welfare, often assumed to have been a much later development. Allbutt was struck off the Medical Register by the General Medical Council, largely because he had published this work at a low price, thus bringing it 'within the reach of the young of both sexes, to the detriment of public morals', but he was not actually prosecuted.[29] Respectable professional men, however, were not immune from the rigours of the law: in 1891 Henry Young, a barrister and a Malthusian, was prosecuted for disseminating the pamphlet *Some Reasons for Advocating the Prudential Limitation of Families* via the Royal Mail, on the grounds that he had distributed it broadcast and that it 'obviously tended to promote illicit intercourse'.[30]

The Malthusian League was wedded to a philosophy of *laissez-faire* individualism and opposition to state intervention. This did not endear it to the British Labour movement, and the subject was largely scorned, partly for its association with these economic doctrines which placed the onus on individual self-help rather than collective action and partly out of a more general moral squeamishness, by socialist parties.[31] The League's philosophical underpinnings increasingly came to appear retrograde and outmoded with the growing involvement of local and central government in health provision from the end of the nineteenth century. This militated against wider acceptance of its doctrines.

From the 1870s the British population began to decline, for reasons which are still debated by historians and demographers. The crude birth rate more than halved between 1871 and 1914. There were various factors inclining couples to restrict their families. Trade was undergoing decline, legislation restricting child labour and enforcing attendance at school made children an economic liability rather than an asset to the working classes, while the higher social classes had increasing expenses in maintaining an appropriate life-style and educating children in a manner suitable to their station in society.[32]

How this decline was achieved is also debatable. The contraceptive devices available were often unreliable and there was much prejudice against using them. Often described in advertisements as 'malthusian devices', they were largely purveyed by commercial manufacturers of dubious scruples (one of the grounds for medical objection was this aura of quackery),[33] although some ideologically-motivated Malthusians, such as J. Greevz Fyssher of Leeds and J. R. Holmes of Wantage (the latter actually imprisoned, a Malthusian martyr) did set up their own contraceptive supply businesses.[34] Devices were expensive and of dubious quality and sellers usually also dealt in abortifacient pills which were seldom of any efficacy in inducing miscarriage (to be effective they would have had to be dangerously toxic). Abortifacient manufacturers additionally increased their profits by subsequent blackmail of women who purchased their pills. In 1898 the Chrimes Brothers and William Brown and Associates were prosecuted for this.[35]

Much prejudice against contraception focussed on the interposition of an artificial device. Some medical authorities, and handbooks of marriage, while deploring 'artificial checks', recommended the avoidance of pregnancy by natural means, principally by having intercourse during the 'safe', infertile period. However, in the extreme ignorance about the mechanism of ovulation which existed, this was entirely misunderstood, and the period usually recommended as 'safe' was what modern calculations of the rhythm method would designate as extremely fertile. The other 'natural' or non-appliance method, coitus interruptus, was considered deleterious to health, and was disliked by many men.[36] Many couples practised total abstention for longer or shorter periods in order to limit their families to what they could afford and the wife's health could bear.[37]

By the end of the nineteenth century there was an active feminist movement arguing for reform in the marriage and divorce laws and increasingly concerned about venereal disease, as well as campaigning for political rights, but it had little enthusiasm for birth control. 'Artificial checks' were felt to encourage the indulgence of male lust rather than protecting the woman's health. However, a few women, such as Alice Vickery (the consort of C. R. Drysdale) and Jane Hume Clapperton of the Malthusian League, did make a feminist case for the employment of contraception. Lucy Bland has recently argued that some writings which have been read as anti-malthusian were deploying a rhetoric about 'restraint' very similar to that of the Malthusian League, and may have been decoded by contemporaries into an advocacy of 'artificial checks', provided these were employed within a ideal and spiritual relationship.[38] In fact the whole debate around women's right to control the number of children they bore and when they bore them may owe an unacknowledged debt to existing malthusian debates. Concern for women's health and the drain of constant pregnancy had been persisting themes in works by advocates of the malthusian gospel since the 1820s. This could be regarded as a purely humanitarian concern, or an extrapolation of the economic doctrine to consider women's health and energies as resources, liable to be outrun beyond what they could sustain by unregulated maternity. They may have contributed a certain subtext to feminist debates on motherhood by choice.

From around 1900 an increasing anxiety was felt not just about the absolute decline in the population but about its quality. This reflected worries to do with struggles both within the British Empire (such as the wars in South Africa), and with competing European and American nations, and led to the emergence of a eugenics movement. This argued that the feckless undesirable poor were breeding prolifically, creating a drain on national resources, while the more desirable classes were not keeping up to strength. There were many critics of the extremely class-biassed attitudes of the Eugenics Education Society, a body which, while deploring differential over-breeding, disdained to advocate or even discuss birth control until well into the 1920s.[39]

A number of unofficial investigations were undertaken into the troubling phenomenon of population decline. In 1907 Sidney Webb, a leading figure in the Fabian Society, published *The Decline in the Birth-Rate*, a survey of family limitation largely among members of or sympathizers with the Fabian Society during 1905-6. In 1911 Ethel M. Elderton undertook a survey at the instigation of the statistician and eugenist, Professor Karl Pearson, which was published in 1914 as *Report on the English Birthrate Part I. England, North of the Humber*. In 1913 the National Council of Morals set up a National Birth-Rate Commission to enquire into the declining population. This had no official status although its intentions were favourably commented upon in Parliament, while its members included Dr T. H. C. Stevenson of the General Register Office and Dr Arthur Newsholme of the Local Government Board, participating with the consent of their superiors in these Government departments.[40]

The Malthusian League continued to be the only body overtly discussing birth control. It thus attracted, for example, feminists interested in the topic who did not necessarily fully subscribe to the official line it still adhered to under the continued leadership of the Drysdale family. A younger generation – C. V. Drysdale, the son of

149

C. R. Drysdale and Alice Vickery, and his wife Bessie – continued to maintain its original high Victorian, liberal, self-help anti-statism, C. V. Drysdale in particular being deeply opposed to socialism, though in the early twentieth century increasing sympathy towards eugenics led to its incorporation alongside their traditional arguments.[41] This anti-collectivist individualist position meant that although the Labour movement might have been considered a natural ally this was far from the case. Even if all socialists did not dismiss birth control as either offensive to respectability or as a palliative for the evils of capitalism which would be obviated by the triumph of socialism, the subject was not included in their agenda. However, there would appear to have been some tentative discussions in certain left-wing groupings, particularly among working class women's organizations such as the Women's Cooperative Guild.[42]

Evidence for the actual practice of 'limitation' in the late nineteenth and early twentieth centuries is ambiguous. Sidney Webb's survey revealed that in most of the marriages there had been some conscious endeavour to keep down the number of offspring. No indication was given, however, of the means by which this had been attempted or achieved. Ethel Elderton's survey suggested that contraceptives were widely available in many areas, propaganda for family limitation was widespread, and many couples were in one way or another restricting their families.[43] Around 1908 Alice Vickery of the Malthusian League became involved in teaching birth control methods to women in Rotherhithe in a somewhat informal setting, through the intervention of Anna Martin, a social worker there.[44] However, it was only in 1913 that the Malthusian League finally did more than argue the theoretical justifications for prudential restraint and family limitation, and issued a practical leaflet of guidance as to methods, *Hygienic Methods of Family Limitation*. It was only supplied to those signing a declaration that they were over 21, married or about to be, and would be responsible for keeping the leaflet out of the hands of young people.[45]

It has often been suggested that the First World War was a factor in the growing acceptance of, and use of, contraception, and that the issue of condoms for the prevention of venereal disease familiarized men with them. This is not the place for an exhaustive account of the lively historiographical debate around venereal disease control in the British forces during this war, but the 'prophylactic packets' some were recommending, but which were very far from being generally accepted, usually contained tubes of calomel ointment for self-disinfection rather than condoms.[46] However, it may be conceded that during the war many men whose upbringing and lifestyles had been relatively sheltered were exposed to men from very different backgrounds and are on record as having picked up various kinds of sexual information, perhaps including contraceptive advice, in informal barrack-room and mess settings.[47]

A major event in the history of British birth control occurred early in 1918 with the publication of *Married Love: A New Solution to Sexual Difficulties* by Marie Stopes, a distinguished woman scientist whose marriage to a fellow botanist had been annulled two years previously on the grounds of his failure to achieve consummation. *Married Love* said little specifically about birth control, but its radiant vision of a fulfilling marital sexual life assumed that couples would and should practice contraception. In *Wise Parenthood*, published later the same year, Stopes gave practical details. Her preferred form of contraception was the rubber vaginal check pessary: this she regarded as preferable on erotic and hygienic grounds to other methods and moreover it put control into the woman's hands, which Stopes, a committed though sometimes rather contorted feminist, believed to be essential. Although she is often claimed, with some justice, to have been a eugenicist in her views, many of her arguments for advancing the use of birth control among the working classes owed at least as much to traditional malthusianism, with her claims for the improved health benefits to mother and child (and by extension to society as a whole) of the smaller, better-spaced, family.[48]

The copious correspondence received by Stopes reveals as does nothing else the moral and practical confusion of contemporary couples trying to limit their families. They complained about the unreliability and unaesthetic nature of the means they had been using. A significant number of couples had been using abstention as the only reliable expedient. Several indicated that while they desired to limit their families, they found 'artificial means' repugnant. There were those who did not dare seek advice from their doctor, and others who had done so to no avail, or even rebuke for daring to mention it. Careful justification was given for seeking Stopes's advice: it was not idle curiosity, they were married, they had already 'done their duty' by producing several children, their state of health precluded further offspring, their resources only just covered the necessities of the children they already had. Many, especially working class women, were desperate for advice, though they frequently assumed that Stopes could do something to relieve them of unwanted pregnancy already under way: she shrank in horror from requests for abortion, prudently enough give the state of the law.[49]

Stopes had been involved with the Malthusian League, but in 1921 held a mass meeting in central London to promote the cause of birth control, which led to the establishment of her own Society for Constructive Birth Control. She presented this as a modern, up-to-date campaigning body putting a positive, rather than a negative, case for the use of birth control, unlike, she almost openly stated, the fuddy-duddy Malthusian League, even though, as can be seen, her own arguments owed a good deal to traditional malthusianism. As she had re-created her own life story,[50] and written out of the narrative the debt she owed to Margaret Sanger for information about the check pessary,[51] she also endeavoured to rewrite the entire history of the British birth control movement to present herself as its pinnacle.[52] She did however remove the freethought irreligious connotations which clung to the advocacy of birth control, associating it with a nondenominational aura of spirituality and indeed claiming, in *A New Gospel to All Peoples*, 1920, to have had a message direct from God to exhort the bishops of the Church of England to give their approval to contraception.[53] In the spring of 1921 she set up in Holloway, a slum district in North London, a 'Mothers' Clinic', the name underlining her commitment to happy and fulfilled maternity.[54] A few months later the Malthusian League established its own clinic in Walworth in South London: again, its title, Women's Welfare Centre, carefully avoided actual mention of birth control. Control shortly passed out of the League's hands. In order to change its image to one more suitable for this new era, in 1922 the Malthusian League renamed itself the New Generation League. In 1925, however, it reverted to the old name, although the journal continued under the title of *The New Generation* and was increasingly independent of the classically malthusian old guard represented by the Drysdales.[55]

Throughout the 1920s the campaign for birth control proceeded on several fronts. Stopes and other reformers believed that contraception should and eventually would be available to the masses via the existing system of maternal welfare centres which formed part of local government public health provision – the voluntary clinics they set up were partly to supply a model and partly to provide information as yet unavailable through other channels. The idea that contraceptive advice should be available 'on the rates' however, received a setback in 1922 when Elizabeth Daniels, a nurse and health visitor, was dismissed from her post in Edmonton for giving birth control advice. The Ministry of Health ruled that this formed no part of the duties of local government public health provision.[56]

1923 was a year of *causes celebres* for the birth control struggle. In January of that year the libertarian communists Guy Aldred and Rose Witcop were prosecuted for publishing, under the imprint of their Bakunin Press, and selling, Margaret Sanger's pamphlet on *Family Limitation*. They had been doing so since 1920 but a new edition seems to have caused worries by its illustrations and vague allusions to abortion. In spite of distinguished names rallying to their defence, the magistrate found the work obscene. Marie Stopes held herself aloof from this, refusing her support.[57] Shortly afterwards she herself made the subject of birth control newsworthy and a topic of polite conversation, to a far greater degree than she had yet achieved with her writings, through her highly-publicized libel suit against Dr Halliday Sutherland. In an anti-birth control tract Sutherland, a Roman Catholic, had described a woman clearly identifiable as Stopes as experimenting on slum women. The case, which went through various stages of appeal, ran for several years and accrued considerable newspaper coverage.[58]

Meanwhile other campaigners were establishing clinics, and endeavouring to persuade the Ministry of Health to withdraw its ban on birth control in publicly-funded welfare centres. Women in the Labour Party set up the Workers' Birth Control Group to achieve this end. Unfortunately in spite of repeated overwhelming votes in support at conferences of Labour women, the Party hierarchy was exceedingly timid, fearing the reaction of both Catholics and Nonconformists. The Malthusian League became involved in these various initiatives, with the rise to influence within it, along with its new identity as the New Generation League, of individuals such as R. B. Kerr and Stella Browne who promoted approaches and alliances previously abhorrent to the Drysdales and the rest of the old guard. Stella Browne was one of the few who spoke up for the potential offered by birth control for women to explore their sexual natures with a freedom previously available only to men, but this radical agenda was very much deprecated by those aiming to influence public policy-making.[59]

The medical profession on the whole maintained its characteristic aloof silence, interspersed with condemnation. Leading medical journals barely mentioned birth control: a brief flurry of correspondence in the *British Medical Journal* in 1921 was followed by nearly a decade of silence on a subject of increasing public and political interest. Women doctors, however, formed an exception to this general rule. The *Medical Women's Federation Newsletter* gave considerable attention to birth control, believing that the subject was one which ought at least to be discussed by medical women. Although eminent lady doctors such as the gynaecologist Lady Barrett or Dame Mary Scharlieb found very little good to say in contraception's favour, younger women doctors, especially those in public health or family practice, were far more enthusiastic and eager to give their patients sound advice, and indeed, to plan their own families. Many sought instruction from Marie Stopes. The subject was increasingly being seen as an issue of maternal welfare, a matter of growing concern at a time when maternal mortality was still high and maternal morbidity widespread.[60]

In February 1927 a Birth Control Investigation Committee was set up, composed of distinguished medical men and scientists, aimed at furthering knowledge of birth control as well as giving it a scientific credibility it had previously lacked. It sponsored research into contraceptive methods, both through scientific research and the systematic collation of data from clinics about their actual practice. Funding for these projects was provided by the Eugenics Society, due to the growing influence within it of a group of younger 'reform eugenists' anxious to dissociate the subject from the old guard's class-biassed rhetoric, and to forge new alliances with the maternal welfare and birth control lobbies.[61] The tide was definitely turning by this year: the leading feminist organization, the National Union of Societies for Equal Citizenship, which had previously held aloof from the birth control campaign, swung its not inconsiderable forces into support of the issue.[62] In August the Malthusian League held a Jubilee dinner: in December C. V. Drysdale declared that the work of the 50-year-old League was complete, as the birth rate had halved since its inauguration and the class fertility differential had diminished substantially.[63] The League however lingered on in a kind of limbo afterlife, without an office or a paid staff or a practical leaflet. Existing members remained as members unless they resigned or died, and the council met intermittently, and indicated that it might occasionally wish to make public pronouncements. The journal *The New Generation*, however, continued to be published.[64]

The terms of the wide-ranging Local Government Act which came into effect in 1929 were capable of the interpretation that local Medical Officers of Health might authorize birth control advice in welfare centres independently of Ministry approval. The Ministry of Health was besought to indicate whether this was correct. As a result, Arthur Greenwood, Minister of Health in the Labour Government, issued Ministry circular 153/MCW in 1930, permitting contraceptive advice to be given as part of post-natal services, to women whose health would be seriously endangered by further pregnancy. This was not generally disseminated, but only sent to local Medical Officers of Health who specifically requested guidance. However, Marie Stopes published a leaked copy in her journal *Birth Control News*, and the newly formed National Birth Control Council, a coordinating body of existing birth control organizations, printed copies and sent them out with an explanatory circular of its own.[65]

The National Birth Control Council shortly afterwards changed its name to the National Birth Council Association, reflecting a constitutional change and a broadening of the parameters of its activities. While continuing to disseminate the circular 153/MCW and to monitor what local authorities were doing about implementing it, the NBCA lobbied for extension of its terms, achieved in 1934 with Ministry circular 1408, broadening the grounds upon which contraceptive advice might be given to include 'other forms of sickness, physical and mental, which are detrimental to them as mothers'. The Association continued to run existing, and to open new, clinics and ran training courses for doctors and nurses.[66]

It produced an 'Approved List' of contraceptives which had been proved by thorough testing and in use to be both safe and reliable.[67] This provided a standard of quality previously lacking in the commercial underworld of seedy 'rubber goods' manufacturers, and its significance should not be underestimated. The industry was so impressed by the marketing potential of a place on the 'Approved List' that some claimed this accolade when it was not merited.[68] Far more people bought contraceptives 'over the counter' than ever attended clinics, and by setting these standards, the NBCA provided more reliable products. Perceiving that most couples who desired to practice contraception did not have access to clinics, the Association opposed attempts to restrict the sale of contraceptives.[69]

The research activities of the NBCA were substantially underwritten by the Eugenics Society, although the NBCA remained cautious about forming too close ties with eugenics. However, its financial resources were limited and they could not spurn this well-off benefactor.[70] Funding was sought by varied means: a 'Malthusian Ball' organized in 1933 may be noted, the name perhaps illustrating the persistence of the term 'malthusian', or possibly its renewed currency following the publication of Aldous Huxley's *Brave New World* with its 'malthusian belts'.[71]

During the 1930s there was considerable, reverse-Malthusian in the classic sense, anxiety over declining population, embodied in such works as *The Twilight of Parenthood*.[72] Partly in this context, and partly in the related context of concern over the continuing high rate of maternal and infant mortality and morbidity, there was also anxiety about the prevalence of induced abortion. The Infant Life (Preservation) Act of 1929 seemed to make a rather ambiguous concession towards the legitimacy of medical judgement in terminating a pregnancy to save the mother's life, but the legal situation was very far from clear. Most abortion was self-induced or performed by amateur 'back-street' abortionists.[73] The Joint Council of Midwifery and the British Medical Association both conducted investigations,[74] and in 1936 a group of veterans of the birth control campaign (mainly the leading participants in the disbanded Workers' Birth Control Group) formed the Abortion Law Reform Association to campaign for legalized abortion under hygienic conditions for women who desired it.[75] In 1938 a government Interdepartmental Committee (the Birkett Committee) was appointed to investigate the subject though no legislation resulted.[76] In the same year Aleck Bourne, a gynaecological surgeon, performed a abortion on a girl of fourteen who had been gang-raped in order to test the law. His defence in court was that although she was in no mortal danger continuing the pregnancy posed a serious threat to her mental health. This established an important case-law precedent under which doctors could legally perform abortions.[77]

In 1939 the National Birth Control Association changed its name to the Family Planning Association, which may partly reflect these anxieties around depopulation, but may also indicate a new ideology of the 'planned family' as central to modernized family values – apparently a very different conception from late nineteenth century 'prudential checks'. But the new Objects of the Association as promulgated in May 1939 began with the classically malthusian statement: 'to advocate and promote the provision of facilities for scientific contraception so that married people may space or limit their families and thus mitigate the evils of ill-health and poverty' (and were conspicuously lacking in any concession to eugenics, in spite of the persistent support of the Eugenics Society towards contraceptive research).[78]

Between the wars the very large family had come increasingly to signify fecklessness, although there was still some obeisance to the idea of fairly large families – or deprecation of small ones – at least among the professional classes. Women doctors responding to a questionnaire about their own use of birth control in 1944 tended to indicate that they would have liked more children but that circumstances had not been favourable. As also mentioned in a questionnaire on their experiences with contraception in their medical practices, the war had provided a considerable deterrent to increases in family size – usually temporary, but in the cases of women who had started families fairly late (as women doctors, like other professional women, would have been likely to do), a permanent halt.[79]

The Royal Commission on Population, which reported in 1949, commented favourably on the work of the Family Planning Association and strongly advocated the benefits of planned spaced families.[80] However, birth control services were omitted from the National Health Service in 1948. Possibly there was a continuing assumption that it was a classically malthusian 'self-help' strategy, an economic expedient rather than an essential element in social medicine. Doctors could advise patients but appliances could not be prescribed except on strictly medical grounds. Medical schools seldom included teaching on birth control in the curriculum and most doctors who wanted to obtain training had to do so privately at Family Planning Association clinics which ran special sessions for this purpose.[81] The Family Planning Association was subject to continuing constraints such as restrictions on advertising. This situation eased when Iain MacLeod, the then Minister of Health in the Conservative Government, played a well-publicized part in its Silver Jubilee celebrations in 1955.[82]

A major development in the contraceptive field was of course the Pill, introduced into the UK in the early 1960s. This was far more popular with doctors than the old appliance methods since it required no specialized training and did not require the doctor to have any intimate contact with the patient's genitals, which fitting the cap had necessitated.[83] Another development of the early sixties, reflecting societal change, was the opening of the Brook Clinics (1964) which gave advice to the unmarried.[84] This decade also saw growing concern – a return of traditional Malthusian anxieties – over global population explosion.[85]

In Britain in 1967 new permissive legislation gave local authorities discretion to subsidize contraceptive supplies.[86] In the same year after much Parliamentary struggle an Abortion Law Reform Act was passed which legalized abortion under medical control in cases where women's physical or mental health was threatened, taking into consideration adverse social conditions (this was somewhat less than the abortion at the woman's choice which the Abortion Law Reform Association had been initially set up to work for). Even before the legislation passed a vociferous anti-abortion lobby had sprung up and agitated for restriction of the law.[87] In 1971 the Lane Committee was set up to enquire into the working of the Abortion Act: it concluded that apart from commercial sector abuses, the Act worked well and as intended.[88] However, attempts to limit and even repeal the law continued over the next two decades. Even so, the law remains substantially the same: if it has not been significantly eroded, neither has it moved in the direction of great liberalization.

Although this surgical operation thus became available free under the National Health Service, anomalously the provision of preventive birth control was still not fully integrated. After several years of campaigning free birth control was inaugurated as part of the new National Health Act of 1974. The Family Planning Association handed over its responsibilities in birth control provision to local Health Authorities, retaining its role in development, training, and education.[89] Shortly after this, the Conservative Secretary of State for Social Services, Sir Keith Joseph, regrettably echoed the eugenic arguments of an earlier era in an appeal for the need to control the reckless feckless breeding of undesirable groups.[90]

To come up to date: in a climate of pressure on resources, specialized birth control clinics have been seen as 'soft targets' for cuts within the National Health Service and eliminated in many areas. Some health authorities no longer routinely perform 'social clause' abortions, for financial rather than ideological reasons.[91] While in theory the preventive work of birth control and the remedial backup of abortion continue to form part of British health services, economic and political realities present a different picture which does not give cause for optimism. Recent anxieties about single mothers echo earlier eugenic concern with 'problem families'. Meanwhile, if there are persisting fears about global over-population, in Britain there is more anxiety over what appears to be a well-established counter-Malthusian pattern, with an inverted pyramid of aging population supported by ever-shrinking cohorts of young.

What, however, is abundantly and enduringly clear from a consideration of the debates over contraception and the evidence for its increasing use in Britain, is a dichotomy between the anxieties expressed in public and the private practices of individuals and couples. Public debates have registered concern over declining population, or a perceived reproductive differential between 'desirable' and 'undesirable' elements within the nation. In private life, however, the choice to restrict family size has almost always been for malthusian reasons, in order to ensure that the actual family did not outstrip the resources available, both the capacity of the mother to bear and rear healthy children whilst preserving her own well-being, and the economic resources necessary to maintain or attain the lifestyle felt to be appropriate.

[An earlier and shorter version of this paper appeared as 'Les mutations de malthusianisme: l'évolution de la perception politique et morale du birth control en Grande-Bretagne', in Francis Ronson, Hervé le Bras and Elizabeth Zucker-Rouvillois, *Demographie et Politique* (Dijon: Éditions Universitaires de Dijon, 1997).]

Notes

1 Roy Porter and Lesley Hall, *The Facts of Life: the creation of sexual knowledge in Britain, 1650-1950* (London and New Haven: Yale University Press, 1995), 65–90.

2 Barbara Brookes, *Abortion in England, 1900-1967* (London: Croom Helm 1988), 22–50.

3 David Gaimster, Peter Boland, Steve Linnane and Caroline Cartwright, 'The archaeology of private life: the Dudley Castle condoms', *Post-Medieval Archaeology* 30 (1996), 129–142.

4 Angus McLaren, *Reproductive Rituals: the perception of fertility in Britain from the sixteenth century to the nineteenth century* (London: Methuen, 1984).

5 Angus Mclaren, *Sexuality and Social Order: the debate over the fertility of women and workers in France, 1770-1920* (New York: Holmes and Meier, 1983), 14–22.

6 Peter Fryer, *The Birth Controllers* (London: Secker and Warburg, 1965), 71.

7 Fryer, *The Birth Controllers*, 71–72.

8 Fryer, *The Birth Controllers*, 43–48.

9 M. L. Bush, *What is Love? Richard Carlile's Philosophy of Sex* (London: Verso, 1998), 8–9.

10 Bush, *What is Love?*, 107–108.

11 Iain D. McCalman, *Radical Underworld: Prophets, Revolutionaries and Pornographers in London, 1795-1840* (Cambridge: Cambridge University Press, 1988).

12 Barbara Taylor, *Eve and the New Jerusalem: Socialism and Feminism in the Nineteenth Century* (London: Virago, 1983), 54–55.

13 Taylor, *Eve and the New Jerusalem*, 215–216.

14 Taylor, *Eve and the New Jerusalem*, 155.

15 Janet Farrell Brodie, *Contraception and Abortion in 19th-Century*

America (Ithaca, NY: Cornell University Press, 1994), 125–130.

16. 'A Graduate of Medicine' [George Drysdale], *The Elements of Social Science; or, Physical, Sexual, and Natural Religion* (London: E. Truelove, 1871, first published 1854), 14–19.

17 Miriam Benn, *The Predicaments of Love* (London: Pluto Press, 1992), 24–9.

18 Benn, *Predicaments of Love*, 10–13.

19 Benn, *Predicaments of Love*, 12–23.

20 Benn, *Predicaments of Love*, 15; Fryer, *The Birth Controllers*, 160.

21 Cited in R. A. Soloway, *Birth Control and the Population Question in England, 1870-1930* (Chapel Hill, NC: University of North Carolina Press, 1982), 117.

22 Fryer, *The Birth Controllers*, 123–131; cutting from *Western Daily Mercury* 28 Nov 1868, South Devonshire Election: scrapbooks, the Amberley Papers, Bertrand Russell papers, McMaster University.

23 S. Chandrasekhar, *'A Dirty Filthy Book': The writings of Charles Bradlaugh and Annie Besant on Reproductive Physiology and Birth Control, and an Account of the Bradlaugh-Besant Trial* (Berkeley, CA: University of California Press, 1981).

24 Fryer, *The Birth Controllers*, 167–169.

25 Benn, *Predicaments of Love*, 164–166.

26 Benn, *Predicaments of Love*, 141–143.

27 C. H. F. Routh, 'On the Moral and Physical Evils likely to follow if practices intended to act as Checks to Population be not strongly discouraged and condemned', *Medical Press and Circular*, 1878 (reprinted in pamphlet form, 1879).

28 Lesley A. Hall, '"The English have hot-water bottles": the morganatic marriage between the British medical profession and sexology since William Acton' in Roy Porter and Mikulas Teich (eds), *Sexual knowledge, sexual science: the history of attitudes to sexuality* (Cambridge: Cambridge University Press, 1994), 350–366.

29 Fryer, *The Birth Controllers*, 169–172.

30 Fryer, *The Birth Controllers*, 172; 'The Post Office and the Malthusian Propaganda: Important Prosecution for Obscenity', cutting from the *Weekly* [?], 17 October 1891, John Johnson ephemera collection, 'Sex, population and eugenics' Box 1, Bodleian Library, Oxford.

31 Soloway, *Birth Control and the Population Question*, 70–90.

32 Simon Szreter, *Fertility, Class and Gender in Britain 1860-1940* (Cambridge: Cambridge University Press, 1996).

33 Angus McLaren, *Birth Control in Nineteenth Century England* (London: Croom Helm, 1978), 221–230.

34 Material on Greevz Fyssher in John Johnson Ephemera Collection, the Bodleian Library, 'Sex Population and Eugenics' box 1; Frank Poller, *Holmes of Hanney* (E. Hanney, Oxon.: Hanney History Group, 1993).

35   Brookes, *Abortion in England*, 4; McLaren, *Birth Control in Nineteenth Century England*, 231–253.

36 McLaren, *Birth Control in Nineteenth Century England*, 125–127.

37 Lesley A. Hall, *Hidden Anxieties: male sexuality 1900-1950* (Oxford: Polity Press, 1991), 91–96; Szreter, *Fertility, Class and Gender in Britain 1860-1940*, 389–424.

38 Lucy Bland, *Banishing the Beast: English Feminism and Sexual Morality, 1885-1914* (London: Penguin, 1995), 189–221.

39 Richard A. Soloway, *Demography and Degeneration: Eugenics and the Declining Birthrate in Twentieth Century Britain* (Chapel Hill, NC: University of North Carolina Press, 1990), 1–17.

40 Porter and Hall, *The Facts of Life*, 183–187.

41 Benn, *Predicaments of Love*, 186–189.

42 Gillian Scott, 'A "Trade Union for Married Women": The Women's Co-operative Guild 1914-1920' in Sybil Oldfield (ed.), *This Working-Day World: Women's Lives and Culture(s) in Britain 1914-1945* (London: Taylor and Francis, 1994), 18–28.

43 Porter and Hall, *The Facts of Life*, 184.

44 Benn, *Predicaments of Love*, 204–206.

45 Fryer, *The Birth Controllers*, 237–239.

46 Lesley A. Hall '"War always brings it on": War, STDs, the military, and the civilian population in Britain, 1850-1950' in Roger Cooter, Mark Harrison and Steve Sturdy (eds), *Medicine and the Management of Modern Warfare* (Amsterdam: Rodopi, 2000), 205–23.

47 Hall, *Hidden Anxieties*, 40–46.

48 Lesley A. Hall, 'Uniting Science and Sensibility: Marie Stopes and the narratives of marriage in the 1920s' in Angela Ingram and Daphne Patai (eds), *Rediscovering Forgotten Radicals: British Women Writers 1889-1939* (Chapel Hill, NC: University of North Carolina Press, 1993), 118–136.

49 Lesley A. Hall, 'Marie Stopes and Her Correspondents: Personalising population decline in an era of demographic change', in Robert A. Peel (ed.), *Marie Stopes, Eugenics, and the English Birth Control Movement* (London: The Galton Institute, 1997), 27–48.

50 Hall, 'Uniting Science and Sensibility'.

51 F. W. Stella Browne to Marie Stopes, 14, 18, 22 Sept 1922, Stopes to Browne, 19 Sep 1922, ms draft 'Attack on the Birth Control News',

Marie Stopes papers in the Contemporary Medical Archives Centre, Wellcome Library for the History and Understanding of Medicine, 'ML-Gen' correspondence, CMAC: PP/MCS/A.42.

52 Norman Himes's correspondence with Marie Stopes, 1926–1928, Himes papers in the Countway Library, Harvard University Medical School, BMS C77 Box 47 folder 538.

53 June Rose, *Marie Stopes and the Sexual Revolution* (London: Faber and Faber, 1992), 136–137.

54 Soloway, *Birth Control and the Population Question*, 208–217.

55 Soloway, *Birth Control and the Population Question*, 183–197

56 Soloway, *Birth Control and the Population Question*, 282.

57 Soloway, *Birth Control and the Population Question*, 230–231.

58 Rose, *Marie Stopes*, 163–175.

59 Soloway, *Birth Control and the Population Question*, 285–303.

60 Lesley A. Hall, '"A suitable job for a woman"?: women doctors and birth control before 1950' in *Women and Modern Medicine*, edited by Larry Conrad and Anne Hardy (Amsterdam: Rodopi), forthcoming.

61 Soloway, *Demography and Degeneration*, 187–188.

62 F. W. Stella Browne, 'Victory – or Compromise?', *New Generation* 6 (1927), 39

63 *The New Generation* 6 (1927), 87; Soloway, *Demography and Degeneration*, 206.

64 Herbert Cuttner of the Malthusian League to Norman Himes, 6 Jan, 8 Oct 1928, 26 Nov 1929, Norman Himes papers in the Countway Library, Harvard University Medical School, BMS C77 Box 34 folder 383.

65 Soloway, *Birth Control and the Population Question*, 308–311.

66 Audrey Leathard, *The Fight for Family Planning: The Development of Family Planning Services in Britain 1921-1974* (London: Macmillan, 1980), 51–59; Soloway, *Birth Contol and the Population Question*, 315.

67 Leathard, *The Fight for Family Planning*, 57.

68 Medical Committee of the NBCA Minutes 13 Jan 1935, Family Planning Association archives at the Contemporary Medical Archives Centre, Wellcome Library, CMAC: SA/FPA/A.5/88.

69 Minutes of the NBCA Executive Committee, 23 Jun 1937, CMAC: SA/FPA/A.5/2.

70 Soloway. *Demography and Degeneration*, 208–213; Lesley A. Hall, 'Women, Feminism, and Eugenics', in Robert A. Peel (ed.), *Essays in the History of Eugenics* (London: The Galton Institute, 1998), 36–51.

71 Leathard, *The Fight for Family Planning*, 56.

72   Soloway, *Demography and Degeneration*, 226–258.

73   Brookes, *Abortion in England*, 27–29.

74   Brookes, *Abortion in England*, 67–68, 70.

75   Brookes, *Abortion in England*, 94–98.

76   Brookes, *Abortion in England*, 105–132.

77   Brookes, *Abortion in England*, 69–70.

78   Leathard, *The Fight for Family Planning*, 68; Soloway, *Demography and Degeneration*, 213–214.

79   Medical Women's Federation archives in the Contemporary Medical Archives Centre, Wellcome Library, CMAC: SA/MWF/J.24/1 'Royal Commission on Population 1945', 1944–1945.

80   Leathard, *The Fight for Family Planning*, 83–85.

81   Hall, '"A Suitable Job for a Woman"'.

82   Leathard, *The Fight for Family Planning*, 93–94.

83   Leathard, *The Fight for Family Planning*, 104–117.

84   Leathard, *The Fight for Family Planning*, 138–147.

85   Leathard, *The Fight for Family Planning*, 177–189.

86   Leathard, *The Fight for Family Planning*, 157–166.

87   Brookes, *Abortion in England*, 154–156.

88   Ashley Wivel, 'Abortion Policy and Politics on the Lane Committee of Enquiry, 1971-1974', *Social History of Medicine* 11 (1998), 109–135.

89   Leathard, *The Fight for Family Planning*, 190–200.

90   Leathard, *The Fight for Family Planning*, 203–203.

91   Porter and Hall, *The Facts of Life*, 272.

8

Reproduction and Revolution:
Paul Robin and Neo-Malthusianism in France

Angus McLaren

In *fin-de-siècle* Europe no nation had a lower fertility rate than
France, yet no nation heaped as much opprobrium on the public
defenders of the practices that resulted in restriction of family size.
The explanation for this apparent contradiction lies in the
bourgeoisie's schizophrenic view of contraception. Respectable
society tolerated it in practise; it opposed it theory. The commercial
opportunities offered by the sale of birth control materials were such
that businessmen with no ideological interest in population control
flooded the market.[1] In the back of the popular sex manuals such as
those produced by the prolific Dr. Jaf were advertisements for
'preservatives' and safety sponges, douching waters like 'l'eau
Cyprienne' and contraceptive sheaths with evocative names such as
'Le Favori' [the Favourite], 'Le Nervi' [the Gangster], and 'Le Cygne'
[the Swan].[2] On offer in Doctor-Brennus's *Amour et securité*, which
first appeared in 1893 and boasted 108 editions by 1906, were
pessaries ('ovule antiseptique') douches, sponges, bidets,
contraceptive powders ('Le Philutérus'), diaphragms ('fosset
utérophite'), vaginal protectors ('L'Infallible'), capuchons ('Bonnet
fin-de-siècle'), baudruches, condoms in a variety of colours and
imitation crocodile hide, as well as a list of 'novelties' including
'ceintures électrique,' 'pommades virginale,' 'anneaus contre la
spermathorrhée,' 'ceintures de chasteté,' and 'serviettes pour
menses.'[3] Moral purity advocates complained that young men were
exposed outside lycées and dances halls, cafés and concerts to a
constant barrage of temptations and seductions of cards,
photographs, newspapers, books stereoscopes and cinematographs.
Boys were offered, in publications that carried advertisements for
'moyens anticonceptionnels' and abortifacients the purchase of
everything from lewd slides to fully inflatable rubber women.[4]

Only when libertarian politics and neo-Malthusian notions were
mixed did the authorities become truly alarmed and that is in fact

what occurred. Those drawn to the public defence of birth control came from the most radical fringes of politics. But with the French birth rate falling in advance of the rest of Europe how could such subversives hope to turn a birth control campaign to their political purposes? To answer this question we can do no better than review the career of Paul Robin – France's first and most famous neo-Malthusian. His arch opponent Jacques Bertillion insisted that any attempt to understand the fertility debate had to include an exploration of 'the dreams that haunt this sick brain.'[5] Paul Robin's views were complex and often contradictory, but much more than mere fantasies. What is so fascinating about Robin and his small band of anarchist followers is that by a process of bricolage they fused Malthusian, libertarian, feminist, and hereditarian notions into a revolutionary ideology that came to be known as French neo-Malthusianism.

Paul Robin's (1837-1912) first ambition was to become a doctor.[6] In fact he began his public life as a teacher in provincial lycées but moved quickly, inspired by positivist and socialist leanings into revolutionary politics during the Second Empire.[7] Forced to abandon both France and his profession, he founded in Brussels with Cesar de Paepe and Eugène Hins the Association positiviste. At the same time he entered the International Working Men's Association. It was because of his involvement with the I.W.M.A. that upon his return to France in 1870 he was arrested and again exiled, this time to England. All his life Robin was to prove to be an irritable, difficult man to work with, partly because of the originality of his ideas. After having quarrelled with Bakunin and his followers on the continent, Robin now found himself equally at odds with Marx and his adherents in London. Marx expelled Robin from the executive of the International in 1871, and he thus found himself momentarily cut off from political activity. It was in this frame of mind that he turned to the study of Malthusian economics. In London a Malthusian League was in the process of being set up by the Drysdale family.[8] Malthus had warned of the dangers of overpopulation but opposed artificial methods of fertility control. The members of the League, espousing what would be known as neo-Malthusianism, revised the master's message; according to them, it was futile to expect wide-scale abstinence, and therefore only by a conscious restriction of family size could the working class hope to assure its prosperity. The League thus sought to fuse its socially conservative economic views with a popular appeal for fertility control. Although the League (thanks to the patronage of the Drysdales), was to be kept in existence for over fifty years, it was doomed to failure. It was hardly surprising that the English working classes, at whom its veiled appeals for fertility control were aimed, found repugnant a doctrine which asserted that the poverty they endured was due not to the failings of the social system but to their own fecklessness.

While the Malthusian League was singularly unsuccessful at home, it did prove itself capable of interesting foreign observers in the population question. This was due in part to the fact that it was tolerant of continental socialists because their theorising posed no direct challenge to English society. The Drysdales' most important convert, a disciple who was to turn the neo-Malthusian message to his own purposes, was Paul Robin. Convinced that fertility control complemented the revolutionary struggle, in 1877 he tried to win the support of the anarchist congress at Saint-Imier; he was rebuffed.[9] He then produced an appeal intended for the 1879 congress of socialists at Marseilles. It was in this way that *La Question sexuelle* was produced, which after revisions appeared as a brochure entitled *Le Secret de bonheur*. In the 1880s Robin had to rein in his enthusiasm for fertility control propaganda. Permitted to return to France by the republican government, he was entrusted by the Ministry of Education, now dominated by anticlericals, with the supervision of an orphanage at Cempuis. Clearly, it would have been imprudent for the director of such an establishment to be known to the public as a sex radical. In any event Robin's nomination to the post was a provocative move in itself. During his years in the International Working Men's Association he had defended the principles of coeducation, the mix of theoretical and practical training known as 'integral education' and positivist morality; at Cempuis he attempted to put this mélange of ideas into practice. He was in later years to be hailed as one of the most important socialist theoreticians of education. Here it is only possible to note that his pedagogical views harmonised with his ideas on population inasmuch as both were founded on the central belief in the rights of individual men *and women* to self-control.[10]

In the 1880s Robin surreptitiously kept up his birth control activities. He visited London for the Malthusian League Conference in 1884 and had Charles Drysdale visit his orphanage in the same year; he used the Cempuis presses to run off copies of *Le Secret de bonheur* and in 1889 opened a Paris dispensary to provide women with contraceptives.[11] There was some talk of these ventures in the press, but it was primarily due to his anticlericalism and defence of coeducation that conservatives succeeded in 1894, during the wave of repression against anarchist outrages, in driving him from his post.[12] Robin later claimed to have been relieved that his new-found freedom permitted him to plunge fully into the fertility debate. He assumed that the time was now ripe for a French version of the Malthusian League; a Dutch neo-Malthusian League had been established in 1885 and a German movement in 1889.[13] Robin himself avoided direct reference to Malthus when he christened his own 1896 organisation the Ligue de la régénération humaine. It had only a small handful of adherents and they came mainly from the ranks of the syndicalist and libertarian left.[14]

The Ligue's first actions were to distribute a birth control tract translated from the Dutch, *Moyens d'éviter les grandes familles* and to set up a journal entitled *Régénération*. Robin himself made direct appeals to doctors, scientists, and politicians for support. Little was forthcoming. Instead, questions were asked in the Assembly about the possible criminality of the Ligue's actions. The popular press expressed its outrage. *Le Figaro* noted that the cartoonist Willette had been prosecuted for a mere caricature and asked why Robin was not tried for his more provocative and perverse 'criminal and immoral propaganda.' *Le Temps* accused him of masquerading as a respectable social observer while undermining the nation, and *La République française* attacked the 'homme de Cempuis' for indulging in bizarre and extravagant theorising that could only weaken the social fabric.[15] Clearly surprised by the violence of the pronatalists' attacks, Robin foolishly responded by asserting that the government was made up of killers and impostors.[16] Threatened with a jail term for this outburst, he fled to London, from which he launched a counterblast, 'Aux richards et aux hommes de lettres.'[17] In the tract he attributed his persecution to the populators and their 'stupid fear of a foreign invasion, and especially, though they do not say it, their terror of the demands of exploited workers.'[18] In failing health Robin decided to remove himself even further from the area of conflict, and in August of 1898 he set sail for New Zealand. For ten months he was befriended by A.W. Bickerton, professor of chemistry and physics at Canterbury College, who at Wainomi had established a commune of sorts called the 'Federated Home.' Bickerton was a feminist interested in questions of fertility control and appears to have provided Robin with additional information on contraception.[19]

Back in France the journal *Régénération* disappeared, but the Ligue did gain the support of one or two radical publications such as *La Fronde* and *Les Droits de l'homme* as well as the adhesion of personalities such as Dr. Adrien Meslier, socialist and future deputy for Paris (1902-1914), J.B. Clément, anarchist poet and editor of the *Petit République*, and Eugène Fourniére, socialist deputy for the Aisne (1898-1902). Assured that he would not be prosecuted, Robin returned to Paris in July of 1899, re-established the Ligue and began again in April of 1900 the publication of *Régénération*. Slowly but surely the organisation built up its support during the next eight years.[20] In fact the Ligue prospered due to its sale of contraceptives and sex manuals. As a result, when a falling-out occurred among the leadership in 1908, with Robin being opposed for his dogmatism by Albert Gros and Eugène Humbert, the movement was not weakened but went on from strength to strength. Gros founded *Le Malthusien* and Humbert *Génération consciente*. Robin, now in his seventies, withdrew from active work, cantankerous as ever, but at least content in the knowledge that he had firmly established a place for the topic of birth control in the population debate.

Why did the public defence of birth control in France become the monopoly of left-wing libertarians such as Paul Robin? To understand how Robin concocted his particular defence of fertility control, it is necessary to disentangle the strands of thought from which it was woven – Malthusian population concerns, degeneration fears, feminist sympathies, and socialist interests. One might begin by noting that there was no shortage of intellectuals in late nineteenth-century France who were explicitly Malthusian and implicitly neo-Malthusian. Charles Drysdale, who attended an 1879 medical congress in Amsterdam, reported that Dr. Leblond of Paris stated that conjugal prudence was not harmful and Dr. Lutaud confirmed the suspicion that most French physicians practised coitus interruptus. Drysdale prevailed upon both to join the Malthusian League's Medical Branch and was also successful in having the economist Yves Guyot and the deputy Alfred Talandier accept posts as vice-presidents of the organisation.[21] What Drysdale could not obtain was the *active* support of these men for birth control propaganda *within* France. Having one's name listed as a corresponding member of a foreign organisation dedicated to the discussion of population problems was one thing; publicly declaring oneself at home an adherent of views which nationalists, alarmed at Germany's higher fertility rates, declared were traitorous was another.[22] Drysdale thus found the neo-Malthusian message propounded in France, not by respectable physicians or social scientists, but by the well-known subversive Paul Robin.

Robin clearly stated in tracts such as *Malthus et les néo-Malthusiens* (1905) that while he accepted Malthus's contention that

169

pressure of population could be a contributing cause of poverty, it was the social system itself which had to be changed. In 1878 he produced the first French work devoted to the defence of fertility control. It was more than this; it was also an attempt to place the notion of the need of the limitation of the size of the working-class family in a political context. The work thus shocked Malthusian economists because of its radicalism while it offended socialists because it linked sex and politics. *La Question sexuelle* began with the ringing appeal:

> Oh, you who are called proletarians (that is to say, makers of children), you who are crushed by an excess of labour, you who are poorly housed, badly dressed, poorly fed, if you sense your pains, if you aspire to things the possession of which would permit you to struggle against the tyranny so well organised by your oppressors, do not burden yourself with a great number of beings more feeble, more powerless than you! Do not encumber yourself with children! . . . Such prudence is as desirable in the daily industrial battle as it is in the violent struggle of the day, very close at hand I hope, of the social revolution.[23]

Whereas the English neo-Malthusians presented birth control as a means by which the poor could adjust to the demands of the capitalist economy, Robin presented it as a measure by which they could prepare themselves for overthrowing capitalism. Technological breakthroughs could be used to free rather than subjugate the masses. He recognised that Malthus had not undertaken his investigations as a disinterested observer but as one determined to destroy the utopian schemes of Godwin and Condorcet. Working-class suspicions of population discussions were therefore warranted. Robin cited as an example the popular poem of Pierre Dupont which included the lines:

> Suivons le peuple et sa science
> Sifflons Malthus et ses arrêts![24]

What the working classes had to be told was that birth control, though not a panacea, was an instrument that could be turned to their own purposes. Priests, economists, and even doctors attempted to keep workers ignorant of their own physiology; some socialists refused to acknowledge the short-term benefits of small families. The real friends of labour would help in the diffusion of contraceptive information so needed by working-class women. Robin was clearly a Malthusian of sorts, but his interests were obviously far removed from the conservatism of both the orthodox Malthusians in France or the neo-Malthusians in England. Though Charles Drysdale helped launched neo-Malthusianism on the continent Robin did not embrace his social conservatism but rather the sex radicalism of George Drysdale whose *Elements* he declared to be the 'Bible' of progressive French neo-Malthusianism.[25]

Robin further distanced himself from English neo-Malthusians by his anti-clericalism and declared suspicion of doctors. He repeatedly attacked confessors, the 'puritards,' and lovingly cited the scabrous exposés of Léo Taxil in such works as *La Bible amusante* and *La vie de Jésus*. In fact many members of the French Catholic hierarchy were doing their best to ignore the national decline in fertility. In the 1890s confessors were advised to be discreet, even after reporting that some parishioners believed everything – especially withdrawal – was permitted in marriage.[26]

Robin expected only the hostility of priests. He initially hoped physicians would back his work and accordingly in 1896 optimistically produced a pamphlet entitled *Aux Docteurs* asking for their help. He insisted that they had the obvious duty of providing a means of contraception that would work even for the negligent. His appeal was met with stony silence. Not receiving the medical profession's support he was soon angrily declaring that doctors were as bad as feminists in asserting that one could rely on abstinence to restrict family size. The sexual continence physicians publicly espoused only confused and made anxious ignorant patients. Robin held doctors responsible for preferring to deal with ill patients than saving them from unnecessary pregnancies. Auguste Forel, the Swiss sexologist, similarly expressed his amazement that doctors, who were happy to discuss prostitution and venereal disease, blushed when dealing with contraception.[27] Bitterly disappointed by doctors' indifference to birth control, Robin attacked them for being happy to deal only with the symptoms of overpopulation such as tuberculosis and alcoholism. Declaring himself now an opponent of the medical monopoly Robin warmly reviewed such anti-medical tracts as Charles Soller and Louis Gastine, *Défends ton peau contre ton médecin* (1902).

Turning Malthusian population preoccupations to revolutionary ends was Robin's first concern; his socialist-feminist interests provided the second important strand in his birth control ideology. Although the leading socialists exhibited a marked lack of sympathy for discussions of gender or fertility, Robin could turn to predecessors on the liberal and anarchistic fringes of the movement for the first hesitant defences of contraception. The nineteenth-century population debate was in part begun because Malthus was jolted into writing *An Essay on the Principle of Population* after detecting in the writings of A.N. de Condorcet (1743-94) an apparent sympathy for artificial methods of fertility control. Referring to the Frenchman's prediction that in the future men and women would control their reproduction, Malthus declared:

> He then proceeds to remove the difficulty of overpopulation in a manner, which I profess not to understand. Having observed, that the ridiculous prejudices of superstition would by that time have ceased to throw over morals a corrupt and degrading austerity he alludes, either to a promiscuous concubinage, which would prevent breeding or to something else as unnatural. To remove the difficulty in this way, will, surely, in the opinion of most men, be, to destroy that virtue and purity of manners, which the advocates of equality, and of the perfectibility of man, profess to be the end and object of their views.[28]

Condorcet had in fact set the line of argument in his *Equisse d'un tableau historique des progrès de l'esprit humain* (1794), which was to be followed by later birth control advocates. He wrote that soon

> . . . men will then know that, if they have obligations to those beings who are not yet here, it consists not of bringing them into existence, but of making them happy; they have for their purpose the general well-being of the human species or of the society in which they live; of the family to which they are attached, and not the childish idea of burdening the world with useless and unfortunate beings.[29]

Condorcet had been one of the few philosophes to subject both gender roles and the family to critical examination. He was not satisfied that either had been predetermined by nature to continue in their present forms, and he thus had no qualms when it came to questioning the value of population growth as a sign of public prosperity.

By his defence of women's right to work in the meetings of the International and by his practical efforts to promote coeducation at Cempuis, Robin gave abundant proof of his concern for women's rights. In his birth control campaign activities he sought to complement Condorcet's stress on the freedom of the woman with the provision of contraceptive information, which might make such freedoms a reality. Robin's first step in this direction was the establishment of a dispensary in Paris in 1889 from which handbills were distributed that proclaimed:

> Mothers of families, young women who soon will be, all you who
> wish to assure yourselves of a lasting happiness, learn what every
> woman should know, consult Mmes L. . . . and Co., teachers of
> hygiene, whose wise opinions are based on the most certain data of
> the science of life and society. You will bless for the rest of your life
> the day of your visit.[30]

In 1895 he followed up this appeal with a series of handbills
including *Aux gens mariés!* and *Femmes, soeurs bien-aimées*. The key
passage of the former read:

> The greatest comfort that one can give to an anxious wife is to
> indicate to her safe, effective means of becoming a mother only
> when she has, after careful reflection, decided to do so. *It is the first
> step, the essential point of the real emancipation of woman*, and in turn
> of the entire race.[31]

And in the latter pamphlet Robin counselled women on their right
to control their fertility.

> This depends on you, you are absolutely the mistresses of your
> destiny. It is necessary that you do not ignore the fact, neither you
> nor your companions in suffering, that science has emancipated you
> from the frightening fate of being mothers against your will.[32]

Tom Laqueur recently reminded us that the notion of sexual
incommensurability was employed by many nineteenth-century
commentators to shore up the belief in fixed gender roles.[33] Given
the notion of separate spheres it was assumed in respectable society
that men would take the initiative in contraception.[34] For countering
such notions Robin was attacked by Passy at a meeting of the Société
d'economie politique. Robin was not without defenders. A woman in
the audience, shocked by the patronising way in which conservative
economists expounded on women's duties, exclaimed, 'They speak
about women at the fireside just as they would speak of the dog in its
kennel.'[35] The pronatalists propounded the image of pampered and
selfish women being responsible for France's fertility decline; Robin
sought to turn attention to the plight of poor women, constantly
fearful of the impact that an undesired pregnancy would have on
their family's well-being.

Robin even dared to moved on from promoting methods of
contraception to defend abortion.[36] Alexander Cohen, a Dutch
anarchist, had in 1895 drawn radicals' attention to the issue by

castigating a British judge who sentenced to death a fifty-seven year old Aston midwife-abortionist. Robin congratulated Cohen on his gallantry and took a growing interest the woman's right to terminate a pregnancy.[37] In response the demographer Arsène Dumont attacked Robin and, while lamenting France's low fertility rate, declared 'it is regrettable that there is a single Frenchman who would congratulate himself for contributing to it [the country's low fertility], who would desire that it is even further aggravated and advocate *surgical means* capable of leading to abortions and a lowering of the birth rate.'[38] The economist Yves Guyot, who had joined Drysdale's Malthusian League in 1877, accused Robin of defending 'preventive homicide.'[39] Robin actually lauded the usefulness of contraceptives as a way of avoiding the risky termination of pregnancies, but he attacked the law against abortion as particularly penalising the poor.[40] Society's murders were, he asserted, worse than any committed by individuals.[41] As far as Robin was concerned what was wrong about abortion – a 'pis-aller' or regrettable last resource – was that at present it was an extremely dangerous undertaking.[42] And that be blamed on the French medical profession which in 1905 he castigated for its cowardly avoidance of the issue. Some doctors secretly provided abortions but that was not enough for Robin.

> For the use of unintelligent, clumsy, poor women doctors should not content themselves with providing abortions in secret; they must energetically defend their natural right to provide them when they are individually and socially useful, and break down the idiotic and ferocious obstinacy of the backward (attardés) who make and apply harmful laws. There might be as a result, though it is not certain, more abortions than now, but they will not pose for the woman more sufferings and dangers than those which today, being clandestine, go wrong (révississent), or for the children, the innumerable attempts that fail.[43]

The medical profession, Robin chided, had to show a little courage.[44]

Robin thus placed the rights of women at the centre of his defence of birth control, providing alternative images to those of motherhood.[45] The first number of *Régénération* in 1896 declared the Ligue's goal to be to 'win for woman the FREEDOM of MATERNITY'.[46] This freedom Robin saw as restricted in the first instance by the teachings of the church that sought to inculcate in women's minds real and imaginary terrors. Even after marriage the woman could find herself subjected to the unfeeling demands of a husband in a relationship that was little better than prostitution.[47]

Sexual intercourse, Robin asserted, was an essential ingredient of a healthy life but could only be fully appreciated by the woman freed by a scientific education from religious prejudices and freed by knowledge of contraception from fear of pregnancy.[48] He believed that at the moment, because such knowledge was lacking, only a small per centage of women found true happiness in marriage. He attacked Léon Blum's *Du mariage* (1907) – a book whose critique of matrimony was regarded by most as daringly subversive – by sarcastically noting that only on page three hundred did the author refer to the impact of child-bearing on family life. Serious readers, Robin insisted, wanted practical advice in place of such sentimental musings.[49] Similarly he complained that feminists spoke vaguely of the woman's 'right to choose the time of maternity,' but prudishly did not say how it would be avoided or postponed.[50]

It is tempting simply to call Robin a feminist but to do so would require ignoring his hostility towards most orthodox members of the women's movement in *fin-de-siècle* France. Indeed he asserted that, 'the word "feminism" is obviously an anti-male battle cry' and he attacked the notion of women being the 'victims' of men.[51] He praised a feminist-socialist like Nelly Roussel but was disdainful of the reformist concerns of most adherents of the women's movement.[52] They, for their part, cautiously avoided discussions of abortion and contraception and were appalled by Robin's defence of prostitution and free love.[53] Even a leftist defender of abortion like Madeleine Pelletier found repugnant Robin's crude assertions that to protect her health every woman had to sexually active.[54]

In making such claims Robin struck a particularly modern note in expressing his concern that the workings of the body be made intelligible to the masses. Given his defence of 'le droit de coït,' his critique of marriage and his assertion that one of the benefits of contraception was that it would allow sexual experimentation, he would appear to warrant the label of sex radical. Like most on the left, however, Robin believed that liberty would not undermine but improve morality. He broke some taboos while accepting others. A common ploy of anarchists – resolute opponents of the state, the church, and the military – was to accuse the elites of being the real immoralists. Some libertarians attributed homosexuality, for example, to the constraints of barracks life. When the Russian fleet visited Toulon a French admiral welcomed it with the unfortunate words, 'Every Russian sailor will have his French sailor, just as every French sailor will have his Russian sailor.'

> Mon dieu! [wryly commented an anarchist writer] we are not
> puritans, and we know that in the army these mores are allowed and
> in common use. And yet is it really necessary to give so much
> publicity to things that cannot do anything for the repopulation of
> France?[55]

As a proponent of co-education Robin had likewise claimed that
vice was cultivated by the sexual claustrophobia of single sex schools
and voyeuristic confessors' tainted enquiries.[56] He believed that a
mixed education in fact prevented sexual precocity; he even sought to
prove this by pointing to a late change in the voices of his charges.[57]
Robin similarly believed that the sexual perversions of adults were a
result of a lack of 'normal' outlets for sexual needs.[58] Wives were
forced to consent to their husbands' demands for 'unnatural' sexual
practices, he asserted, because they did not have access to
contraceptives.[59] If an unmarried man could not lead an active
heterosexual life he might become faut de mieux a homosexual.
Oscar Wilde, victimised as he was by hypocritical moralists, was
defended by French anarchists but this did not prevent Robin and
others from condemning bourgeois society as decadent and
presenting themselves as the champions of a reinvigorated
heterosexuality.[60]

A third element clearly discernible in Robin's defence of birth
control was his concern about degeneration.[61] The hope that the
rational control of fertility could aid in the improvement of the race
was implied in the title Robin gave his organisation–Ligue de la
régénération humaine. Even his earlier educational activities revealed
how much he had been marked by his scientific interest in Darwin
and Comte. At Cempuis he kept careful anthropometric records on
his charges, at the same time allowing them every freedom. In a
curious way he thus manifested a hankering after positivistic
certainties combined with a love for Fourierist spontaneity.[62] This
same tension could be found in his defence of birth control. On the
one hand he defended contraception on libertarian grounds, but on
the other he spoke of the *duty* of the handicapped to limit their
fertility. In the writings of the English neo-Malthusians there was also
a strain of eugenic thinking based on the fear that the better sort were
in danger of being out-bred by the inferior. Indeed, Francis Galton,
the father of eugenics, and most of his closest followers were of the
opinion that the main impact of birth control had been negative in
nature inasmuch as it had been practised mainly by those who owed
it to the community to reproduce. The task posed modern society

was to limit the breeding of the inferior and sponsor that of the superior.

Such eugenic arguments did not make much headway in France at the turn of the century, partly because the French were still loyal to Lamarckist notions of acquired characteristics and not as given to talk of racial stock as were the English and Germans. Georges Vacher de Lapouge, the anti-Semitic follower of Arthur de Gobineau, did discuss in *Les Séléctions sociales* (1896) the relationship of racial purity to fertility and concluded that miscegenation was the root cause of France's low rate of natality, but his bizarre theories attracted few adherents.[63] More down to earth were the concerns expressed by Dr. Auguste Lutaud writing under the pseudonym 'Dr. Minime' in 1891 in the *Journal de Médecine de Paris* on 'Le néo-Malthusianisme'. Citing Bertillon's figures on the 1886 census of Paris, Lutaud pointed out that the wealthiest quartiers had the lowest birth rates and the poorest, the highest. The 'degenerate' produced as a consequence a disproportionately high percentage of the next generation. In self-defence the nation would, he argued, have to propagate among the poor methods of contraception while attempting to win the wealthy back to the traditionally large family.[64]

Robin had no desire to increase the family size of the wealthy and he certainly did not view the working class as a threat. In using the term 'degenerate' he was thinking not just of the 'unfit' but of prolific Catholics and foreign labourers. The terminology was vague enough, however, for Robin to use the issue in the 1890s as part of his initial attempt to seek to win the support of the socially respectable. In 1896 he appealed in such terms to the Société d'anthropologie de Paris and later recapitulated his argument in a brochure entitled *Dégénérescence de l'espèce humaine: causes et remèdes*. The gist of his argument was that natural selection no longer effectively removed weak stock.[65] Thanks to advances in medicine and hygiene, those who might once have perished could now survive. Natural selection no longer worked, indeed due to medical advances saving the weak reverse selection now took place.[66] If a better society were to be created, Robin asserted, the state could not support forever an increasing burden of misfits; the only sensible solution was to adopt a policy of what he referred to as 'le méliorisme,' by which the genetically weak would be provided with the means to avoid offspring through either contraception or sterilisation.[67] His goal was a world in which the individual would be assured a good birth, a good education, and a good social organisation.

Robin's point was that France already had a low fertility rate so the task was to reduce that of the worst – the 'inférieurs' or 'tarés.'[68] There was an obvious sad irony in a revolutionary envisaging the sterilisation – perhaps with Rontgen rays – of the mad, epileptic, deaf, bald, myopic, tubercular and the poorly sexually developed.[69] In France most vocal defenders of sterilisation were those alarmed by the prospect of social unrest.[70] How Robin hoped to square his libertarian views with his hereditarian concerns was never made clear, but two points raised by the issue must be stressed. First, Robin was far from being the only one on the left tantalised by the notion of improving the race. The hereditarian message attracted mainly turn of the century progressives who saw in science a way of creating a meritocracy, but it also drew important numbers of reformers and revolutionaries imbued with the positivistic belief that no aspect of social life was immune to scientific improvement.[71] Second, Robin was neither a racist nor an anti-Semite. His companions-in-arms consisted of those very anarchists, vagabonds, ex-convicts and prostitutes that the respectable – following criminal anthropologists like Cesare Lombroso – customarily condemned as the archetypical degenerates.[72] Robin took a perverse pleasure in turning the fear of degeneracy argument against the respectable and to the purposes of advancing the revolution.

A preoccupation with the advancement of socialism formed the fourth and final strand in Robin's fertility control ideology. The socialist and anarchist rank and file ultimately provided him with his main support. The leading lights of both movements were not impressed by Robin's arguments, however, and asserted that birth control had become his hobby-horse, his 'dada.' He did not deny it.[73] Birth control, he claimed, had to be viewed as a tactic worthy of revolutionaries' interest because of the attacks made on it by priests, generals, capitalists, chauvinists – all the 'procréatomanes.'[74] In addition Robin held out the hope that fertility control could play some role in strengthening labour by restricting the employer's access to large numbers of workers; the birth strike or 'grève de ventre' could be made part of the tactic of the general strike.[75] At the very least the self-conscious use of contraceptives could be viewed as an example of the anarchists' vaunted 'propaganda by the deed.' And lastly Robin warned that since the victory of birth control was inevitable, it would be to the left's discredit if it were not numbered among its supporters. 'It would be a pity for the history of official socialism that it [the victory] occurred *despite* it. It is already bad enough that our successes until now have been obtained *without* its support.'[76]

From the turn of the century until 1908 Robin's indefatigable efforts made the subject of fertility control a topic of national debate. The message carried in *Régénération* was more or less an elaboration of Robin's views on neo-Malthusian economics, degeneration, feminism, and socialism. The Ligue's main concerns were to win as many influential recruits as possible and to provide practical contraceptive information to the masses. By 1900 when an international meeting of neo-Malthusians was held in Paris, the Ligue could count as supporters not only J.B. Clément, Eugène Fournière, and Adrien Meslier but also Dr. Lapique of the Sorbonne, Dr. Alfred Naquet, the influential socialist and 'father of French divorce,' and Charles Malato, editor of *L'Aurore*.[77] *Régénération* appeared monthly carrying reports of Robin's lectures, which were usually held in bourses du travail, the local union halls. In his work he was assisted by new recruits: his son-in-law Gabriel Giroud, the feminist Nelly Roussel, and, most important of all, the young anarchist Eugène Humbert.[78]

To avoid prosecution under the law against 'les associations philosophiques,' Robin's Ligue proper had to consist of less than twenty persons associated for the purposes of publishing the journal. Such precautions were necessary. Those associated with the Ligue's activities were, because of their involvement with anarchists, subject to police surveillance and occasional prosecution. In 1900 the secretary-treasurer of the Ligue was fined for distributing a birth control tract; in 1901 Sicard-Palange was prosecuted in Bordeaux for selling Robin's *Santé de la femme*; in 1904 the *Réveil syndical* of Lens was similarly tried for printing a neo-Malthusian article; in 1906 a certain Émile Hamelin who was distributing both anti-militarist and Ligue material was arrested in Trelazé; in 1907 Victor Cornil, the Ligue representative in Roubaix, was prosecuted, and in 1908 Dr. Fernand Elosu, another anarchist-pacifist, was jailed for two months in Bayonne for selling *L'Amour inféconde*.[79]

Such persecution served only to further radicalise the French neo-Malthusians. Typical of the Ligue's propagandising efforts was the discussion of birth control held at a meeting of the Union syndical du bronze at the Paris Bourse du travail on June 23, 1903.[80] The speakers included Charles Desplanques, Auguste Liard-Courtois, 'Libertad' (Joseph Albert, the founder of *L'Anarchie*), V.J. Gelez, and Mme. Louise Reville. It was in the ranks of the syndicalists that the Ligue found its most active supporters, but the working-class audience was more interested in practical information than in abstract theorising. When the speakers drifted too far afield, they were interrupted by cries of 'Les moyens!' To respond to such demands the Ligue sold tracts such as *Aux femmes, Aux gens mariés,* and *Moyens d'éviter les grandes familles* for fifty centimes, Allbutt's *Le livre de l'épouse* for one franc, and Drysdale's *Eléments de science sociale* for three francs fifty.[81] Those who sought personal information were informed by the journal that consultations were offered by medical practitioners whose addresses would be provided on demand.[82] Advertisements were carried in *Régénération* for a variety of condoms, both the soluble and Mensinga pessaries, douches, douching solutions, and bidets. Detailed information was also provided on how douching was to be carried out, how primitive condoms could be made from animal intestines, and how soluble pessaries could be prepared at home. Concerning the latter, Robin provided a recipe for a 'pâté préservative' consisting of gelatine, glycerine, and quinine, a mixture which he insisted produced a product as reliable as the commercial brands of pessaries.[83] Robin's concern was to make information concerning contraception and sexuality in general as accessible as possible to the working class. He was interested in every form of contraception. In his old age he was even attacked as a satyr by *Le Malthusian* for purportedly trying to test the notion that if one conscientiously massaged a woman's breasts she could be kept artificially lactating and thus provided with a natural form of contraceptive protection.[84]

It was by the sale of contraceptives that the Ligue made much of its income. It is hard to think of any other revolutionary group which could boast – as Robin's did – that it made money from selling goods meant to subvert the state. The provision of contraceptives was not only monetarily rewarding; it complemented the anarchists' desire to win a degree of self-sufficiency for the workers.[85] The fact that the English Malthusian League did not provide such services was commented on by Giroud in 1910. 'The English propagandist leaves the responsibility of the diffusion of neo-Malthusian appliances to merchants.'[86] The French activists saw themselves as playing some part in overthrowing the existing economic system whereas their English counterparts had no such desires.

This essay began by noting the apparent contradiction of the French bourgeoisie embracing fertility restriction while publicly opposing it. By cutting through the rhetorical excesses of both the neo-Malthusians and the pronatalists, it is made clear that they shared a number of concerns – both sides found the issues of differential fertility, degeneration and the purported rise of the perversions worrying. As far as the bourgeoisie was concerned, it is likely that – despite the protests of pronatalists like Bertillon – few found the anarchists' demographic ideas particularly preoccupying; what the respectable found alarming was Robin's 'sick dream' of turning population theories – whose genealogy could be traced back to Thomas Malthus – to the purposes of inciting revolution.[87] The two groups chiefly differed on the question of agency. The French neo-Malthusian anarchists – inciting their labouring audiences to control their own destinies – used the issue of the workers' right to contraception as a basis for cultural resistance to the state. They were so vociferous because fertility was already being brought down by the elite. Everyone knew that the upper classes employed contraceptives themselves but, asserted Robin, through shameless hypocrisy they used appeals to morality, decency, and national need to prevent their being obtained by those who most needed them.

The bourgeoisie called for social responsibility; Robin and his followers for individual freedom. The French bourgeoisie, carefully limiting its own family size, by its hypocritical silence left the public defence of contraception to the libertarians. One is reminded that in the 1830s English pornography was largely produced by radical printers because the Vice Society – in driving such publications underground – necessarily restricted their production to those skilled in avoiding prosecution and imprisonment.[88] Similarly the French pronatalists in asserting the disreputable nature of the public defence of contraception allowed it to be monopolised by the anarchists. The latter eagerly turned to subversive purposes the poor's demands for such information. A fierce opponent of Robin, the criminologist Alexandre Lacassagne became famous for his epigram, 'Societies have the criminals they deserve.'[89] What he and other prontalists failed to note was that French society was similarly fated to produced in the person of Paul Robin the radical neo-Malthusian it merited.[90]

Notes

1. Jean-Pierre Bardet and Jacques Dupâquier, 'Contraception: Les français les premiers, mais pourquoi?' *Communications* 44 (1986), 3-33.
2. Dr. Jaf, *Amour et mariage en Orient* (Paris: J. Fort, 1908).
3. Doctor-Brennus, *Amour et securité* (Paris: C. Chollet, 1895); Doctor-Brennus, *Histoire du célèbre ouvrage: amour et securité* (Paris: F. Montel, 1895).
4. Emile Pourésy, *La Gangrène pornographique* (Roubaix, Foyer Solidariste, 1908), 214-37; Alexandre Lacassagne, *Peine de mort et criminalité* (Paris: Maloine, 1908), 89-91.
5. William Schneider, *Quality and Quantity: The Quest for Biological*

Regeneration in Twentieth-Century France (Cambridge, Cambridge University Press, 1990), 35.

6. He entered the Ecole de médicine navale in 1855 but left for the Ecole normale in 1858.

7. On Robin's life see Gabriel Giroud, *Paul Robin* (Paris: G. Mignolet et Storz 1937); Christine Demeulenaere-Douyère, *Paul Robin (1837-1912): Un militant de la liberté et du bonheur* (Paris: Publisud, 1994); Francis Ronsin, *La Grève des ventres: Propagande néo-malthusienne et baisse de la natalité française* (Poitiers: Aubier Montaigne, 1980), 42–93.

8. See Rosanna Ledbetter, *A History of the Malthusian League, 1877-1927* (Columbus: Ohio State University Press, 1976) and Angus McLaren, *Birth Control in Nineteenth Century England* (London: Croom Helm, 1978), 107-113; Richard Allen Soloway, *Birth Control and the Population Question in England, 1877-1930* (Chapel Hill, University of North Carolina Press, 1982), 55-69.

9. James Guillaume, *L'Internationale* (Paris: Société nouvelle de librairie et d'edition, 1905), 4:223; Giroud, *Robin*, 22-25.

10. On Cempuis see Gabriel Giroud, *Cempuis* (Paris: Schleicher frères, 1900); Dr. Henri Fischer, *De l'education sexuelle* (Paris: Ollier-Henry, 1903), 175-80; and Angus McLaren, 'Revolution and Education in Late Nineteenth Century France: The Early Career of Paul Robin', *History of Education Quarterly* 21 (1981), 317-335.

11. *National Reformer* (July 1884), 58; *Malthusian* (July 1884), 538; (October 1893), 73; (May 1895), 35.

12. *Malthusian*, July 1895, 50-51; Giroud, *Robin*, 88.

13. Hugo Röling, '*De tragedie van het geslachtsleven': Dr. J. Rutgers (1850-1924) en de Nieuw-Malthusiaansche Bond (opergericht 1881)* (Amsterdam: Van Gennep, 1987); James Woyke, *Birth Control in Germany, 1871-1933* (London: Routledge, 1988), 38, 54; Cornelie Usborne, *The Politics of the Body in Weimar Germany* (London: Macmillan, 1992), 6-9.

14. *Malthusian* (June 1896), 45.

15. *Le Figaro* (13 January 1897), 1; *Le Temps* (11 January 1897), 1; *La République française* (15 January 1897), 1.

16. On pronatalism in France see P. E. Ogden and M. M. Huss, 'Demography and Pronatalism in France in the Nineteenth and Twentieth Centuries', *Journal of Historical Geography* 8 (1982), 283-98; Hervé Le Bras, *Marianne et les lapins: L'obsession démographique* (Paris: Orban, 1991); Joshua H. Cole, "There are Only Good Mothers': The Ideological Work of Women's Fertility in France Before World War I', *French Historical Studies* 19 (1996), 639-72;

Jay Winter and Michael Teitelbaum, *The Fear of Population Decline* (New York: Academic Press, 1985).

17. On Robin's account of the events of 1897 see *Régénération* (April 1900 and January 1903). See also the special flyer of the summer of 1897 put out by *Régénération* in which it was asserted that the Darlan-Béranger bill against outrages against morality was aimed at the Ligue.

18. *Malthusian* (October 1898), 75. Robin cited Leygoens, Cornely, Lombelins, and Bertillon as responsible for his persecution. See also *Le Gaulois* (11 January 1897), 1; Giroud, *Robin,* 233–34.

19. Robin reported in *Régénération,* April 1908: 'I saw in the Antipodes ingenious housewives who made for themselves for a derisory price an object having the same efficacy as the best brands of pessaries, ovules, cones...'. Bickerton – apparently influenced by Max Nordau – had organised a curious commune of about thirty people living in tar paper shacks and producing fireworks. See R. M. Burdon, *Scholar Errant: A Biography of A. W. Bickerton* (Christchurch: Pegasus Press, 1956), 69-70; see also *Malthusian* (April 1899), 26, 36-37; (June 1899), 42; (July 1899), 50.

20. It was reported in 1904 that the Ligue had a thousand subscribers and about twenty sections. See *Malthusian* (February 1904), 9.

21. Alfred Talandier was also an honorary vice-president of Bradlaugh's Secular Society; see *Malthusian* (October 1879), 69; (April 1883), 408.

22. On French views of the Malthusian League see 'La Ligue Malthusienne: son origine et son histoire', *Journal des économistes* 11 (1880), 241-248; Pierre Mille, 'Le Néo-Malthusienne en Angleterre', *Revue des deux mondes* 108 (15 December 1891), 911-928. The French so associated the English economist with the notion of fertility control that the term 'malthusianiser' was coined to describe family restriction.

23. Giroud, *Paul Robin,* 24-25.

24. Paul Robin, *Malthus et les néo-Malthusiens* (Paris: Librairie de Régénération, 1905), 3.

25. Paul Robin, *Le Néo-Malthusianisme* (Paris: Librairie de *Régénération,* 1905), 2; George Drysdale's *Physical, Sexual and Natural Religion* (London: Truelove, 1855) appeared in French as *Les éléments de science sociale* (1869).

26. Martine Sevegrand, *Les Enfants du bon Dieu: Les catholiques et la procréation au XXe siècle* (Paris: Albin Michel, 1995), 25. *L'Ami du clergé* spread the pronatalist message, yet called for discretion. The clergy were divided, the French bishops remaining silent on the issue until 1919.

27. Auguste Forel, *La Question sexuelle* (Paris: Steinheil, 1911), 491.
28. T. R. Malthus, *An Essay on the Principle of Population* (London: J. Johnson, 1798), 154.
29. Antoine-Nicholas de Condorcet, *Esquisse d'un tableau historique des progrès de l'esprit humain*, O. H. Prior (ed.) (Paris: Boivin, 1933), 222–23.
30. Giroud, *Robin*, 209.
31. Giroud, *Robin*, 214.
32. Giroud, *Robin*, 214.
33. Tom Laqueur, *Making Sex: Body and Gender from the Greeks to Freud* (Cambridge, Mass.: Harvard University Press, 1990).
34. Anne-Marie Sohn, *Chrysalides: femmes dans la vie privée (XIXe-XXe siècles)* (Paris: Publications de la Sorbonne, 1996), II, 818-20
35. *Malthusian* (March 1897), 17-18.
36. James M. Donovan, 'Abortion, the law and the juries in France, 1825-1923', *Criminal Justice History* 9 (1988), 157-88; Sohn, *Chrysalides*, II, 828-908.
37. See the letter of Cohen on 20 November 1896 from the Amsterdam jail to Kaya Batut about his meeting Robin at the 1896 International Socialists Workers and Trade Union Congress in London. I owe this reference to Ronald Spoor who is editing Cohen's letters. On Cohen's defence of abortion which appeared in *The Torch of Anarchy*, (18 December 1895), 107 and was reprinted in the American journal *Rebel*, February 1896, 56 see Angus McLaren, *The Trials of Masculinity: Policing Sexual Boundaries, 1870-1930* (Chicago, University of Chicago Press, 1997), 81–84.
38. *Bulletin de la société d'anthropologie de Paris*, 7 (1896), 142.
39. *Malthusian* (October 1896), 73.
40. *Régénération* (October 1903), 208; (November 1903), 221; (March 1904), 239. See also Rachel Fuchs, *Poor and Pregnant in Paris: Strategies for Survival in Nineteenth Century France* (New Brunswick, Rutgers University Press, 1992).
41. *Régénération*, (July 1903), 183–4.
42. *Régénération*, (July 1905), 58.
43. Paul Robin, *Le Néo-Malthusianisme* (Paris: Librairie de *Régénération*, 1905), 18–19.
44. On the feminist and medical discussions of fertility control, see Jean Elisabeth Pedersen, 'Regulating Abortion and Birth Control: Gender, Medicine, and Republican Politics in France, 1870-1920', *French Historical Studies* 19 (1996), 673-98.
45. Elinor A. Accampo, 'The Rhetoric of Reproduction and the Reconfiguration of Womanhood in the French Birth Control

Movement, 1890-1920', *Journal of Family History* 21 (1996), 351-71.

46. *Régénération* (December 1896), 1.

47. Robin, *Le Néo-Malthusianisme*, 7-10; and see also Paul Robin, 'La Question de néo-Malthusianisme', *Revue de morale sociale* (1903), 202-203.

48. Robin went so far in his sex radicalism as to assert that the way to improve the lot of prostitutes was not by 'rescuing them – but by organising them'. He believed that in the long run reliable contraception by permitting greater sexual freedom would put an end to prostitution; in the short run he saw prostitutes fulfilling an unfortunately necessary role though one in which they risked their health and indeed their lives. Accordingly the task was to protect as much as possible women who were as virtuous as many wives, not by police regulation which only created pimps and extortion, but by the unionisation of women for their own self-defence. Robin advanced his views in *Propos d'une fille* but because of police hostility his hopes of establishing a *Ligue anti-esclavage* and a journal, *Le Cri de filles*, came to nothing. See Giroud, *Robin*, 164–5. Fittingly Octave Mirbeau, who married a prostitute, was a defender of Robin. See Octave Mirbeau, *L'Amour de la femme vénale*, tr. du Bulgare Alexandre Levy (Paris: Des femmes dans l'histoire, 1994).

49. *Régénération* (July 1907), 267.

50. *Régénération* (September 1903), 202-3.

51. *Régénération* (August 1905), 67; and on 'Vrai féminisme' see *Régénération* (January 1907), 213-4; (March 1907), 232.

52. On Roussel see Accampo, 'The Rhetoric of Reproduction', 356-63.

53. Karen Offen, 'Depopulation, Nationalism and Feminism in Fin-de-Siècle France', *American Historical Review* 89 (June 1984), 648-76.

54. Claude Maignien and Charles Sowerine, *Madeleine Pelletier, une féministe dans l'arène politique* (Paris: Editions ouvrières, 1992), 88 and see also Joan Wallach Scott, *Only Paradoxes to Offer: French Feminists and the Rights of Man* (Cambridge, Harvard University Press, 1996), 135-55.

55. Félix Fénéon cited in Joan Undersma Halperin, *Félix Fénéon: Aesthete and Anarchist in Fin-de-siècle Paris* (New Haven, Yale University Press, 1988), 250.

56. Paul Robin, *Sur l'enseignement intégral* (Paris, 1872).

57. *Bulletin: L'Orphelinat Prévost*, September-October 1892, 125; Maurice Dommanget, *Paul Robin* (Paris: Editions S.U.D.E.L., 1952), 32.

58. *Régénération* (September 1902), 103.

59. Giroud, *Paul Robin*, 156.

60. His French defenders included Octave Mirbeau and Félix Fénéon. See Octave Mirbeau, 'A Propos du 'Hard Labour'' in *Les Ecrivains, 1885-1910* (Paris 1926), 39-44.

61. On French intellectuals' preoccupation with degeneration, see Robert Nye, *Crime, Madness and Politics in Modern France: The Medical Concept of National Decline* (Princeton, Princeton University Press, 1984)

62. See McLaren, 'Paul Robin', *passim.*

63. G. Vacher de Lapouge, *Les sélections sociales* (Paris: A. Fontemoing, 1896).

64. Reprinted as Dr. Minime, *Le Néo-Malthusianisme: lettre à M. Max Hausmeister* (Paris: Bureau de publications du *Journal de médecine,* 1891). See Drysdale's warm review in *Malthusian* (January 1892), 4–5.

65. See Robin's speech reported in *Bulletin de la société d'anthropologie de Paris,* 7 (1896), 139-40, 143, 210-212, 224; and also *Régénération* (November 1905).

66. Paul Robin, *Dégénerescence de l'espèce humaine: causes et remèdes* (Paris: P.V. Stock, 1896). Paul Robin, *Le Néo-Malthusianisme* (Paris: Librairie de *Régénération,* 1905), 4.

67. *Malthusian* (April 1896), 25-27; *Régénération,* December 1896. 3.

68. *Régénération* (December 1896), 3.

69. *Régénération* (November 1905), 86-7. For attacks on Robin's eugenicist views expressed at the Congrès de l'assistance familiale in October 1901 see *Régénération* (May 1902), 78-9.

70. Hippolyte Laurent, *Les Chatiments corporels* (Lyon: Phily, 1912), 122-348-50; Antoine Wylm, *La Morale sexuelle* (Paris Felix Alcan, 1907).

71. See Michael Freeden, 'Eugenics and Progressive Thought: A Study in Ideological Affinity', *Historical Journal* 22 (1979), 645-672.

72. E. Fourquet, 'Les Vagabonds criminels', *Revue des deux mondes* 2 (1899), 399-437; Gabriel Tarde, 'Les Crimes de haine', *Les Archives de l'anthropologie criminelles* 9 (1894), 241-54.

73. *Régénération* (August 1903), 195.

74. Paul Robin, *Population et prudence procréatrice* (Paris: Humbert, 1902), 4.

75. Robin, *Population et prudence procréatrice,* 6; *Régénération,* March 1903, 151-2.

76. Robin to Vandervelde (25 January 1903), cited in Giroud, *Robin,* 137. See also *Régénération* (July 1902); April 1903.

77. On the meeting see *Malthusian* (September 1900); *Régénération* (January 1901). *Régénération* also noted the propaganda campaigns

outside of France such as those of the Drysdales in England and Ida Craddock, Emma Goldman, and Moses Harman in America. Quebec, because of its high birth rate was cited frequently as a negative example of the dangers of overpopulation. The report of land being given by the provincial government to large French-Canadian families elicited the response, 'Ca, c'est plutôt bébête'. For other sneering references to 'lapinisme canadien' see *Régénération* (July 1907) and *Génération consciente* (October 1910).

78. Roussel made a first appearance in April 1903, Humbert in March 1903 with an article on 'la grève de ventre', and Desplanques in June 1903 with an essay 'Ayez peu d'enfants' in which he declared that workers needed 'les coudes franches pour la lutte'.

79. On prosecutions see *Régénération* (May 1901); (April 1906); *Génération consciente* (15 July 1908); *Malthusian* (September 1900); *Gazette des Tribunaux* (23 July 1910), 662–3.

80. See a report of the meeting in *Régénération* (August 1903). The syndicalist press also spread word of Robin's activities. *Régénération* listed as papers friendly to the cause and willing to reprint propaganda: *L'Ouvrier coiffeur, Réveil des mécaniciens, Le Combat de Levallois-Clichy, Le Relieur, L'Ouvrier métallurgist, L'Ouvrier syndiqué* (Marseilles), *L'Emancipation* (Toulon), *Réveil syndical* (Lens), *Voix du peuple, Réveil de l'esclave, L'Idée socialiste* (Lyon), *Le Jura socialiste, Le Progrès* (Le Havre), *L'Insurgé* (Liege), *Le Travailleur syndiqué* (Montpellier), *L'Action ouvrière* (Bordeaux), *Le Combat* (Bordeaux), *Petit république* (Paris), *L'Action* (Paris), *Cri de quartier* (Paris), *La Cravache* (Rheims).

81. See *Régénération* (December 1896). In 1905 the Ligue also began to distribute a series of gummed propaganda labels to be stuck on walls. A typical one read:

    L'Avortement est dangereux.
    La prévention de la grossesse.
    est facile et sans danger.
    AYONS PEU D'ENFANTS

82. *Régénération* (April 1908). In *Controverse sur le néo-Malthusianisme* (1905) Robin listed the practitioners to be consulted but – possibly for legal protection – warned, 'Requests for abortion will not be replied to'. Those listed included Dr. Adrien Meslier, Dr. J. Darricarrère, Marot (herboriste), Mme. H. Piens (sage-femme), M. et Mme. Eugène Humbert, Mme. Petit (sage-femme), and other 'pharmaciens' and 'aide-pharmaciens'.

83. The concern for the expense of contraceptives was noted in a cartoon of Alphonse Lévy showing a working woman looking at a

shop window display of preventives and exclaiming, 'Ca, c'est trop cher pour moi'. *Régénération* (February, 1902).

84. *Le Malthusien*, (November 1910), 185–7. *Le Malthusien* under the editorship of Albert Gros began its life carrying attacks against the dictatorial policies of Robin.

85. *Génération consciente*, (May 1912); (April 1914).

86. *Génération consciente* (September 1910).

87. By 1908 disagreements over the employment of the funds (which were in a state of confusion as a result of Robin's anarchistic disregard for the niceties of bookkeeping) as well as the desire of some younger men to throw off the heavy-handed leadership of the old libertarian, led to the break-up of the Ligue. Robin withdrew from active campaigning, and *Régénération* disappeared to be replaced by two competing journals, *Le Malthusien* and *Génération consciente*. Paul Robin ended his life by taking chlorohydrate of morphine, dying 3 September 1912. Giroud, *Robin*, 253-260; *Le Malthusien*, December 1912, 389. On the subsequent history of neo-Malthusianism in France see Roger-Henri Guerrand et Francis Ronsin, *Le Sexe apprivoisé: Jeanne Humbert et la lutte pour la contrôle des naissances* (Paris: La Decouverte, 1990); and on fertility discussions see Françoise Thébaud, *Quand nos grand-mères donnaient la vie: la maternité en France dans l'entre-deux-guerres* (Lyon: Presses Universitaires de Lyon, 1986); Mary Louise Roberts, *Civilization Without Sexes: Reconstructing Gender in Postwar France, 1917-1927* (Chicago: University of Chicago Press, 1994).

88. Iain McCalman, *Radical Underworld: Prophets, Revolutionaries and Pornographers in London, 1795-1840* (Oxford, Clarendon Press, 1988).

89. Henri Souchon, 'Alexandre Lacassagne et l'école de Lyon', *Revue de science criminelle*, 35 (1974), 533-59.

90. For an overview see Angus McLaren, *Sexuality and Social Order: The Debate over the Fertility of Women and Workers in France, 1770-1920* (New York: Holmes and Meier, 1983).

9

Biology and Sociology of Fertility. Reactions to the Malthusian Threat, 1798–1933.

Antonello La Vergata

Nature against Malthus

Historians of Malthusian controversies often forget that these debates were not limited to demographic, economic and statistical issues, but involved broader philosophical and moral concerns over the harmony of nature. Indeed, they often took place on the plane of theodicy and natural theology. Before Malthus, population phenomena were usually seen as part of the balance of nature. Malthus acknowledged that he had cast 'a melancholy hue' over man's hopes for progress but presented his law as an aspect of a providential, though stern, arrangement calculated to stimulate man's higher faculties through exertion and struggle against evil.[1] No wonder, therefore, that, in spite of his pessimism, some of his supporters saw his law as part of natural equilibrium. But, at the same time, to some of his early opponents it seemed only too natural to appeal to the harmony of nature or providence to exorcize the spectres of overpopulation, vice and misery.[2] This holds true not only of popular writers and well-wishers of mankind, but of some economists. Some of them, like the French Frédéric Bastiat, the German Friedrich List and the American Henry Charles Carey, had a nearly mystical belief in universal laws of harmony and in the equilibrium between population and food supply.[3] Also population statisticians were frequently influenced by some belief in the benevolent intent of nature (or God). They looked for regularities, which could easily be interpreted as manifestations of (divine) harmony[4].

An antidote to Malthus's dire forecasts was provided by the widespread belief that fertility spontaneously adjusted itself to varying conditions. In this argument, there was no real danger of overpopulation (or of depopulation). Some authors said unmistakeably that this self-regulation was due to social and psychological factors affecting behaviour and the will.[5] Others, however, tended to attribute it to some sort of physiological mechanism. But very often no distinction at all was made between social and physiological causes. Many contented themselves with pointing out that particular ways of life or social conditions (for instance luxury or urban conditions) influenced the birth rate, without drawing a line between the psychological and the physiological effects of those factors. It was quite common to find such diverse factors as race, age, wealth, occupation, ambition, diet, class, disease, and so on listed without discrimination.[6] And many statisticians were only too happy to accumulate evidence of population trends, and to treat them mathematically, without enquiring into their causes.

Luxury, for instance, had long been pointed out as a cause of declining fertility, and statistics showing the tendency of aristocratic families to fade away were quickly made. But was it luxury as such or the physical consequences of the debauchery it might entail that was responsible for this trend? Towns were often described as noxious places; indeed some went so far as to call them, in Rousseauian terms, 'graves of mankind'.[7] But were they so because they tempted their inhabitants into immoral preventive practices or because those dissipations, polluted air and bad food physically perturbed the generative system? The same questions could be asked concerning virtually all the factors that were thought to reduce fertility (like, for instance, lack of healthy exercise, overeating, alcoholism, nervous strain, and so on). Not until the twentieth century did it become universally clear that even people actually starving or seriously ill might be prolific. Even early theories relating a rise in the standard of living to reduction of fertility left it unclear whether the latter was due to an intensification of prudential restraint or to contracting dangerous physical habits. As late as the 1930s something as difficult to define as 'mental' or 'nervous strain' was alleged by some demographers and economists as a cause of infertility[8]. But it was seldom explained whether this occurred by enfeebling sexual desire, diverting energies from the organs of reproduction to the brain, inducing impotence or reducing the quantity of spermatozoa in seminal liquid. Ambiguity, as is well known, has its appeal. Doctors, reformers, social prophets and moralists wallowed in it for centuries.

An instructive instance of the no man's land where psychological and physiological factors merged into one another – and one which deserves further study by historians of medicine and sexuality – is provided by the long-standing belief that food influences fertility.[9]

Physicians and writers on hygiene kept recommending a healthy, moderate, not too refined diet, alleging as evidence of its good effects the fact that 'the poorest and most laborious Part of Mankind are the fruitfullest'.[10] But there was more at stake than that. Dietary prescriptions were moral as well as medical measures. They were on a par with sermons on chastity and sobriety. Moral (and immoral) practices did not only influence the destiny of the soul, but also altered the body itself. Immoral behaviour impaired its functioning, whereas moral behaviour enhanced physical well-being. The healthy body could not but be the virtuous body. The degree of fertility was the reward for virtue as much as a test of sexual vigour. A 'chain of providences' linked with one another virtue, health, sex, food and fertility.[11] The moral economy of nature was mirrored in the wisdom of the body. This had an important implication: the good functioning of the body, including fertility, was in the individual's hand. As Dr. Richard Price, the pioneer of demography, put it in a passage quoted by Malthus himself in the first edition of the *Essay on the Principle of Population*,

> Were there a country, where the inhabitants led lives entirely natural and virtuous, few of them would die without measuring out the whole period of present existence allotted to them; pain and distempers would be unknown among them; and the dismission of death would come upon them like a sleep, in consequence of no other cause than gradual and unavoidable decay.[12]

The failure, both in scholarly and in popular writings, often to distinguish between psychological and physiological factors was reflected in the confusion between the terms 'fecundity' (the reproductive capacity) and 'fertility' (the actual number of children produced).[13] It is difficult to say exactly when a clear-cut distinction was introduced, still less when it became commonly accepted. The Scottish doctor James Matthew Duncan made a differentiation as early as 1866:

> By fertility or productiveness I mean the amount of births as distinguished from the capability to bear [...] By fecundity I mean the demonstrated capability to bear children; it implies the conditions necessary for conception in the women of whom these variations are predicated [...] In short, fertility implies fecundity, and also introduces the idea of number in progeny; while fecundity simply indicates the quality without any superadded notion of quantity.[14]

191

However, the two terms were often used interchangeably until the 1940s.[15] It was only in 1934 that the Population Association of America officially endorsed the distinction.[16] As a biological capability, fecundity can be altered only by causes affecting directly the reproductive system (accidents, diseases, alterations of physiological cycles). But its actual expression, fertility, can be influenced by social, psychological or behavioural factors eventually leading to a limitation of births. No clear-cut distinction between the two could be generally accepted as long as it was believed that even psychological and behavioural factors, too, could *directly* alter the functioning of the reproductive system. Alcoholism, for instance, whether it was thought to be socially or biologically caused, was long believed to have hereditary effects, because it damaged germ cells. Well into the twentieth century, the range of factors thought to be able to influence the reproductive system was much wider than we think today. Many people believed in some form of inheritance of acquired characters even after this doctrine was challenged by August Weismann in the 1880s. Also non-Lamarckian students of inheritance often attributed a biological basis to characters which we now consider to be overwhelmingly determined by social factors. The eugenics literature contains many striking instances of this lingering tendency to 'biologize' cultural traits.[17]

The confusion between fecundity and fertility, and between biological and cultural factors, played an important role in Malthusian controversies. It led many opponents of Malthus's to believe they could appeal not only to morals and economics, but to a much more powerful ally: the natural laws governing the human body. Nature itself was on their side. Theories proliferated in which the movement of population was deemed to be subject to laws of nature ensuring a beneficent equilibrium. They reflected a growing naturalistic propensity to bring human behaviour in line with that of other living beings. But they also reflected the assumptions of eighteenth-century natural theologies which saw evidence of a providential arrangement of the cosmos both in population phenomena and in the nature of minerals, plants and animals. In stressing the infallible order of nature, nineteenth-century naturalism often took on providentialist tones.[18] Faith in Nature simply replaced faith in God. Indeed, the context in which a great part of the debate over fertility took place could be described as both providentialist and naturalistic.

Malthus's opponents claimed that the providential character of the true law of population lay in its flexibility. As the educationalist, reformer and editor of the *Westminster Review,* William Hickson, put it, 'the ratio of fecundity is variable with circumstances, and not fixed'.[19] Whether they believed that fecundity varied inversely with the 'exertion of mind',[20] with the density of population,[21] with the natural length of the cycle of lactation,[22] or with the abundance of food,[23] these authors wanted to vindicate God's (or Nature's) ways to man, by showing that fecundity was regulated by some self-adjusting law, which at times increased population, while at others reducing it before positive checks become necessary. Physiology was the instrument of the *vis medicatrix naturae.* God's (or Nature's) providential arrangement was implemented through the gonads. Prostitutes were often thought to become sterile as a result of their profession, but to reacquire fertility if they resumed a more moral and healthy sexual life.[24]

Spencer's law

The best known example of a theory of population based on these physico-moral assumptions is the doctrine of the natural antagonism between 'individuation' and 'genesis' Herbert Spencer formulated in 1852 and restated in the second volume of his *Principles of biology* (1867): as the output in the individual's energy used in maintaining life and in personal development increases, the amount of energy available for reproduction decreases; and, conversely, what one puts into reproduction takes away from the individual. For sperm cells, nerves and brain contain the same basic chemical substance, 'neurine', and the healthy functioning of the system depends on a balanced use of it. Thus, 'intense mental application, involving great waste of the nervous tissues, and a corresponding consumption of nervous matter for their repair, is accompanied by a cessation in the production of nerve-cells'. Conversely, 'undue production of sperm-cells involves cerebral inactivity. The first result of a morbid excess in this direction is headache, which may be taken to indicate that the brain is out of repair; this is followed by stupidity; should the disorder continue, imbecility supervenes, ending occasionally in insanity'.[25] But in order to combat the struggle for life resulting from population pressure, people have to apply their intelligence and moral sense strenuously; this brings on an enlargement of these qualities, and a strengthening of the nerves and the brain, which, in turn, lead to the establishment of higher, less fecund human types, until a final stage is reached, when 'the pressure of population [...] must gradually bring itself to an end': 'no more than a normal and pleasurable activity' will be necessary, and 'the obtainment of subsistence and discharge of all the parental and social duties will require just that kind and that amount of action needful to health and happiness'.[26]

Spencer's law, or some sister doctrines, circulated widely until well into the nineteenth century. It was taken seriously by authors as diverse as the philosopher and psychologist Wilhelm Wundt and the socialist leader August Bebel in Germany, the philosopher Alfred Fouillée, the influential psychologist Théodule Ribot and the economist Charles Gide in France, the botanist Alphonse de Candolle in Switzerland, and the biologist Edwin Ray Lankester, the sexologist Havelock Ellis and the eugenicist Caleb Saleeby in England.[27] Its success was due to the fact that it reinvigorated faith in the *vis medicatrix naturae* and provided people of various opinions and political leanings with an anti-Malthusian argument based on the very nature of things: the laws of nature ensured a spontaneous solution of the problem of population.

Like Providence itself, Spencer's law could, and was, used for many different purposes, some of them, as we shall soon see, perversely at variance with his political ideas. The conservative economist and social critic William Rathbone Greg confided that one day 'physiological influences or laws' would be discovered that would prove Malthus to be wrong: 'Providence will be vindicated from our premature misgivings when we discover that there exist natural laws, *whose operation is to modify and diminish human fecundity in proportion as mankind advances in real civilization, in moral and intellectual development*'.[28] Greg was also one of the first to warn against 'the multiplication of the race from its least elegible specimens, or, as it has happily been termed, the non-survival of the fittest'.[29] In civilized nations, he claimed, where the action of natural selection was suspended, the fertility of the educated, healthy and laborious classes was held in check 'by greater providence and more developed brains'.[30] In order to prevent the multiplication of the unfittest, the State should exercise 'a salutary but unrelenting paternal despotism, and supply the deficiency [of restraint] by vigilant and timely prohibition', as well as by mitigating the fertility of the poor by lifting their cultural level.[31] A conclusion hardly consonant with Spencer's advocacy of unrestrained *laissez-faire*, and, after all, with Greg's own faith in natural providence.

The liberal economist Walter Bagehot, too, found an antidote against Malthus' pessimism in the belief that compensating mechanisms operated in nature to obviate social evils. Although he recognized that physiological causes influencing fertility could hardly be separated from other causes such as moral norms, he took it for granted that 'the nervous condition', education and 'the habit of using the mind' reduce reproductive power, especially in women. In the female constitution there is a limited amount of force, and if it is invested in some way, it cannot be used in another. In man the influence which reduces fertility is exerted not so much by mental activity as by strain, anxiety, nervousness, and that kind of higher intellectual work which causes 'a subtle and obscure pain'. Bagehot did not share Spencer's optimistic view of a final stage of equilibrium, but neither did he agree with pessimists like Francis Galton. The race could be deteriorating, as Galton feared, but the reduced growth of urban population seemed to be nature's remedy for the diminished vigour of that population. Great cities are painful spectacles, but 'we can regard them as a huge cleansing machinery, which, no doubt, shows us a great deal that is detestable, but also takes away much of it, and prevents more coming, not only in that place but in others'.[32]

If 'the remedy of pressure and the hope of progress alike lie in advancing individuation', the Scottish biologists Patrick Geddes and John Arthur Thomson argued, 'the practical corollaries of the Spencerian principle, although Mr Spencer can hardly be said to have insisted upon these, are individuate and educate'.[33] This could be done by bettering the environment (material, mental, social, moral) and the organism by 'the conscious and rational adjustment of the struggle into the culture of existence', that is by replacing natural with artificial selection. The two authors went so far as advocating 'artificial preventive checks to fertilization'. It is remarkable – they commented with involuntary irony – that Spencer did not proceed to a fuller application of his principle.[34] A less Spencerian conclusion could hardly be imagined.

But Spencer was to be offered a much more serious occasion to complain: some socialists enlisted him in their army.

Socialists

Although socialism meant many things to many people, it may safely be said that socialists generally detested Malthus. Utopian socialists, Russian populists and Marxists shared in this antipathy.[35] They agreed that the world would support far more people under one system of production and government than another, and that social progress would better the relationships between men, thereby mitigating the consequences of multiplication. In short, man would behave differently in a better society. His nature would to some extent change. He would acquire a greater capacity for rational control over both his environment and his animal appetites. For instance, if mankind was organized so as to devote itself to creative labour and study, the sex instinct would lose much of its appeal.[36] A further check to overpopulation would arise from the higher status of women and their full participation in social and intellectual life. These ideas was in tune with the traditional moral belief that the control over the reproductive instinct was a triumph of reason over instinct. Curiously, this was very much in the spirit of Malthus himself, who made much of man's dignity. But while Malthus had appealed to a moral effort and sacrifice on the part of the individual against his nature, his opponents argued that the same results could be reached, thanks to nature, by a cooperative effort, if not by a smoother and more pleasurable process.

A streak of providentialistic naturalism was particularly evident in French utopian socialists. In Fourier's reorganisation of society, for instance, overpopulation would be prevented by the increased production made possible by the new social order, by contraceptive practices and by four other factors: 1) *la vigueur des femmes* (strong and healthy women being 'more apt for pleasure, but less for conception'); 2) the 'gastrosophic régime' (good food causing a decrease of fecundity); 3) 'phanerogamic customs' (free love being legal, a plurality of lovers will operate as an obstacle to fertility); 4) the integral exercise of all corporeal faculties (a balanced gymnastics for the whole body and a healthy manual work will lead to a slower development of sexual organs).[37]

For Proudhon, too, in the new society there would be a higher harmony between the earth and mankind, and a freer and fuller use of our faculties. Work would inevitably become a more intense and noble activity, which would in turn entail a weakening of fertility.

> The industrial faculty is exercised only at the expense of the prolific faculty [...] Labour is for love an active cause of inertia [...] It affects simultaneously the mind and the body [...] Chastity is the companion of work [...] Men of meditation, energetic thinkers, all great workers are of but mediocre capacity in the service of love [...] Now, if by a necessary law we become ever better at work than our fathers were, it is likewise necessary that we acquire ever *moins de vaillance* in love games.[38]

Proudhon subsequently modified his theory of the antithesis between work and love, and added chastity to labour and study as a factor that would diminish sexual attraction. In a society based on justice, he said, man would be free of the 'fatalism of the flesh'; he would yield to love 'only under the excitation of the ideal'; being engaged in higher pursuits, he would find continence less distracting and sweeter than sexual gratification. By participating in social and intellectual life, women would lose their aptitude for maternity: their *vertu prolifique* and their amorous inclination would cool alike, just as now love of children tend in both sexes to purge conjugal life of eroticism.[39]

Marx and Engels did not indulge in providentialist naturalism. They did not base their rejection of Malthus on optimistic views of future sexuality. They spurned general theories of population based on sociological or psychological factors unconnected with economic ones. They attacked Malthus as a plagiarist, a serf of the ruling classes and an enemy of the poor. Engels poured scorn on his doctrine as 'a monstrous blasphemy against nature and mankind'.[40] Marx stated that overpopulation is a consequence of historical situations, not a law of nature: 'Every special historic mode of production has its own special laws of population, historically valid withis its limits alone. An abstract law of population exists for plants and animals only, and only in so far as man has not interfered with them'.[41] The law peculiar to the capitalistic mode of production is rooted in the nature of capitalistic accumulation, which constantly produces a relatively redundant population of labourers, that is a population of greater extent than suffices for the average needs of the self-expansion of capital. Being more rapid than the increase of variable (or working) capital, the increase of constant (or fixed) capital and its accumulation in the form of production goods lead to less need for labourers, as goods tend to take their place. 'The labouring population therefore produces, along with the accumulation of capital produced by it, the means by which itself is made relatively superfluous, is turned into a relative surplus population; and it does this to an always increasing extent'.[42] Only under these conditions is it true that 'poverty seems favourable to generation', as Adam Smith said. For this amounts to saying that 'not only the number of births and deaths, but the absolute size of the families stand in inverse proportion to the height of wages, and therefore to the amount of means of subsistence'. This law 'calls to mind the boundless reproduction of animals individually weak and constantly hunted down'.[43] 'Accumulation of capital is, therefore, increase of the proletariat'.[44] For the capitalistic system encourages the formation of a large 'disposable reserve army of labour'. Overpopulation is 'a necessity of modern industry',[45] and an adjustment to the social need for a 'rapid renewal of the generation of labourers'. 'This social need is met by early marriages, a necessary consequence of the conditions in which the labourers of modern industry live, only by the premium that the exploitation of children sets on their production'.[46]

Marx's hate for Malthus obliged him to claim that Darwin, whom he greatly admired, was wrong when he said that he had applied Malthus's law to plants and animals: the gist of Malthus's doctrine, Marx said, was that it could *not* be applied to plants and animals, which cannot produce any means of susistence. As a result, Marxists have since then tended to evaluate Darwin and Malthus separately.[47]

It was in a social Darwinist context that attempts were made to find a compromise between Malthus and socialism. A Darwinist long before he became a Marxist, Karl Kautsky accepted Darwin's struggle for life: 'It will last', he said, 'as long as the universe itself, nor will it ever be possible to suppress it: what we can do is to transform the struggle of all against all into the struggle of all for all [that is against nature]'. This was a very common idea among socialist and reformist Darwinists, who saw cooperation as the highest form of the universal struggle, and the only one worthy of man. As a committed Darwinist, Kautsky felt he had to reckon with Malthus. He knew that his opinion differed from that of Marx and Engels, as well as those of other leaders such as Bebel and Liebknecht. Kautsky agreed that Malthus' social doctrine was distasteful and reactionary, but insisted that overpopulation was a real threat – even for the socialist society – and struggle for life was an eternal phenomenon. Indeed, the problem of the spatial limits to human expansion would be aggravated in a socialist society by a better distibution of wealth, which would encourage multiplication and cause a population boom; and this, in turn, could frustrate all progress already made. Kautsky advocated birth control ('conjugal onanism' and 'preventive intercourse'). Moral restraint was a folly, as it led to monstrous evils: sex was necessary to a healthy and virtuous life. Contraception was an essential part of the struggle of man against nature. Kautsky warned his comrades against too great confidence in the self-regulation of things. The appeal to harmony was a typical trick of anti-socialist rhetoricians and apologists of *laissez faire*. It was typical of them to find compensations everywhere. But socialists had to stick to the 'mechanical view of the universe'. Therefore, Kautsky thought it necessary to refute, one after another, the physiological theories of population equilibrium, including those of Spencer, Sadler, Doubleday, Fourier, Spencer, Trall, and Carey (with the latter he had flirted for a while). The idea of a self-regulation of population movement was 'a paroxysm of teleological thinking'.[48]

Kautsky's book probably enjoyed a greater fortune in Italy than in Germany.[49] The French socialist Benoît Malon singled it out to the politician and economist Napoleone Colajanni: Malthus, he said in a letter of 31 March 1880 to his Italian comrade, 'is a first-class scoundrel' and 'his formula is certainly anti-scientific, because it takes a transitory stage of society as the definitive one', but 'his advice of prudence is not to be neglected, especially in Italy'.[50] Colajanni agreed: Malthus was wrong, but his appeal to prudential restraint was a sound one. There can be no absolute overpopulation, but only a relative and artificial one, which is due to ignorance, technological backwardness and bad social organization. Cooperation and altruism must replace animal struggle in human society, but the biological fact of reproduction is 'the elementary, propelling force of economic revolutions as well as historical ones'.[51] Population pressure is the proximate cause of progress, but the further progress of society will control it. A conclusion reminiscent of Spencer, whom Colajanni admired, and whom he, like many Italian socialists, considered as a sort of socialist *manqué*.[52] However, Colajanni did not endorse wholeheartedly the 'most welcome hypothesis' that population is curbed spontaneously. 'The whole of the biological hypothesis [of population movement] lacks so far statistical and really inductive basis', as the facts that confirm it are as numerous as those that refute it. Better, therefore, to rest on firmer ground, and to recommend the 'preventive check', by which Colajanni meant contraception.[53]

Strange though it may seem, welcoming Kautsky's Malthusianism (or, to be more exact, neo-Malthusianism) did not mean abandoning Spencer. A more or less watered down version of Spencer's law became a part of the response of many Italian socialists to Malthus. The socialist leader Filippo Turati is a case in point. He was even more enthusiastic in his appraisal of Kautsky's attempt to amend and absorb Malthus in a socialist framework. It was necessary, he said, to separate 'the reactionary and decrepit Malthusianism of Malthus' himself and of the conservatives from the 'young Malthusianism, positivist and democratic'. 'With this distinction', he went on to say, 'Malthusianism [...] will become the best and necessary ally of democracy and justice, and the only – if the word can still be used – religion of the future'. In Kautsky's book, he wrote, 'is consummated, in the bridal chamber of science, the marriage of Malthusianism and democracy, the one powerless without the other'.[54] For Turati, science included Spencer's law, which apparently complemented that of Malthus: 'Self-restraint, although inefficacious today as a general remedy, could be beneficial in some particular cases. But we hardly believe in sermons. Once the standard of living and the mentality of the poor classes are improved, these classes, too, will become less prolific. Both physiology and psychology are warrants for it'.[55] Turati's combination of Spencer and Malthus squared with his general view of the relationship between social and natural science. Like so many of his colleagues, he wished a reduction of social and economic phenomena to their physical basis (to 'laws as sure and infallible as those of mechanics')[56], and he appealed to the spirit of science to denounce the illusory and 'subversive' faith in man's power to alter things at will: by this he alluded to anarchism, syndicalism and revolutionary Marxism (in fact, some syndicalists, in Italy and in France, argued that family size should not be limited, as a high birth rate would depress wages and hasten the revolution).[57] If socialism had to be scientific, it had to reckon with the laws of nature, including that of 'the eternal antagonism between overpopulation and well-being, in the present and in the future'. Economics could become a science like physics if it recognized a system of laws independent of human free-will. This search for physical, 'fatal' laws of history and economics also inspired Kautsky's translator, Leonida Bissolati. He acknowledged that 'the excess of population is an *artificial* excess, that is, a product of the present economic constitution',[58] but at the same time it was necessary to warn socialists against the 'natural' excess of population that would be possible with the constitution of socialist society. Almost alone among his comrades, Bissolati considered abortion as a means of both birth regulation and women's liberation.[59]

Other Italian socialists seem to have turned to Spencer as a result of their dislike of contraception. Among them was the economist and politician Francesco Saverio Nitti, author of a book which enjoyed great success and was translated into French and English. 'The solution of the problem of population', he wrote, 'which has been scarcely ever anything better than utter darkness to the economist, is to be found in the biological theory, which, conceived by Doubleday, afterwards perfected by Darwin, and precisely formulated by Spencer, has revealed new horizons to demographic science'.[60] 'Biology', he went on to say, 'has revealed the close connection between the birth-rate and the anatomical and phychological progress of mankind'.[61] To the followers of the individualist school who used Spencer's law as a natural sanction for absolute freedom of competition, Nitti replied that quite the contrary was the case: 'A perfect and general individualism will be possible only when the social, not the natural causes, of inequalities shall have been suppressed. The maximum of individuation will, therefore, be possible only in the maximum of socialisation'. Until then, opportunities for individuation will be available only for the rich.[62]

But Kautsky was to change his mind. His 1880 book, he later confessed, was the work of a 'callow young man who understood nothing of Marxism'. So he felt obliged to revise it. As a result, he published another book in 1910, in which he concluded that Malthus was wrong not only with respect to man, but with respect to plants and animals. His law was no natural law at all.[63] Instead, Kautsky praised Spencer's theory of the equilibrium between destructive and conservative forces in all organisms as one of the few scientific theories of the previous century which still stood confirmed.[64] Spencer's explanation, however, failed in many cases. For instance, in women who take an interest in 'the possibility of enjoyment and creativity in nature, art and science', fertility declines 'not because of any physiological mechanism, but because the new woman's higher status will make contraception more appealing to her'.[65] Morality will be the regulator of population in the socialist society. Public opinion and the sense of the individual's duty towards society as a whole will dictate what to do each time population growth varies from the optimum. Then it will be possible to set the basis for an effective, morally-inspired racial hygiene or 'social eugenics'.

In spite of Kautsky, contraception remained 'the especial *bête noire* of socialists, land reformers, and other advocates of redistribution in democratic control'.[66] And, conversely, most neo-Malthusians were anti-socialist. The opposition to neo-Malthusianism and family planning was carried over from democratic to totalitarian socialism. Planned parenthood was seen, at best, as a mere palliative which hindered the real solution of the problem[67] or, at worst, as a bourgeois pseudo-solution imbued with the anti-human nature of capitalist ideology.[68]

Depopulation

Between Kautsky's first and second books, the whole context of the debate on population changed dramatically. A falling birth rate was by now evident in almost all Western countries. Concerns about depopulation replaced the preoccupation with overpopulation. In England, for instance, the birth rate, which was close to 35 per 1000 in the 1840s, began to diminish steadily in the 1880s – with a drop of 10 to 15 per 1000 in some London districts – and by Queen Victoria's death had fallen to 28.5.[69] As man power was generally perceived as the bedrock of State power, and a necessary condition for race expansion, a growing literature on the declining birth rate gave popular currency to talk of national calamity, inevitable decline and race suicide consequent on flagging reproductive energies. That France was in an even worse predicament was, of course, no source of consolation for the British (nor did the French like the privilege of being the champions of *dénatalité* and the harbingers of a declining phase in the history of Western civilization). The alarm in France originated in the 1850s, but reached its climax after 1870. This had important consequences, showing conclusively (at least in some eyes) that Malthus was wrong, and leading to a change in the attitude of French economists towards the population problem. Demographic research and doctrines were inextricably bound with concern for the decline of the country. Between 1800 and 1850, in a France where population was dense and poverty widespread, Malthus' ideas had been favourably received by late physiocrats and liberal economists. In their hands, Malthusianism became an integral part of a broader doctrine of individual responsibility. However, French Malthusians were generally more optimistic than Malthus: they believed in some version of man's perfectibility and thought it possible and advisable to diminish population pressure by teaching people the need to exercise prudence, caution, industry, foresight and thrift. A few of them went so far as to advocate *coitus interruptus*. The general pro-Malthusianism which prevailed between 1800 and 1850 (and which in turn had replaced the pro-populationism of mercantilist writers), gave place to a new populationism.[70] This was accompanied by a loss of faith in the self-regulating character of the laws of nature, by an increasing emphasis on the need for State intervention, and by a growing realization of the cultural and psychological nature of the ultimate checks to fertility. As the philosopher Guyau put it as early as 1887, 'French sterility is much more an economic phenomenon than a biological phenomenon [...] In sum, the question of French population is purely and simply a question of morals'.[71]

Depopulation became a source of national anxiety. Loss of power, prestige and even national identity under the pressure of foreign immigrants seemed imminent. France's defeat in 1871 was interpreted as the fate a nation with a declining birth rate would suffer at the hands of a more prolific and virile race. France had to be remade, Emile Zola declared in his novel *La débâcle* (1892). In many of his later writings, and especially in the novel *Fécondité* (1899),[72] he urged his fellow countrymen to give up selfish pursuits and to perform their sacred duty towards Life and the Country.

For all his faith in the power of inherited tendencies to physical and moral degeneration (which formed the backbone of his Rougon-Macquart series of novels), Zola seemed by the time he wrote *Fecondité* to have shifted towards a more morally oriented interpretation of social issues. His diagnosis of the French disease can be summed up in one word: 'egoism'. Whether be believed that this egoism, which made people in every class (but especially in the rich bourgeoisie) shrink from the danger of encumbering themselves with a baby was itself the result of a biological as well as a moral degeneration, is not clear. There are hints that Zola knew and approved of some version of Spencer's law, but the main thrust of his plea was based on moral and social categories. Love of luxury, social emulation, competitive spirit, hedonism, careerism and so forth led people to embrace 'practical Malthusianism' and to forget their duty towards the country and nature. In Zola's passionate, overflowing, obsessive rhetoric, patriotism merges with the celebration of Life and 'the sacred duty of generation'. However, it is only the healthy that can hear the call of Life and France. They welcome each newborn baby as an unmixed blessing, because they can physically afford doing so. But such is not the case with the morally flawed. Maternity is good for the body of the beautiful and virtuous Marianne, but it has devastating effects on the body of her selfish, plain cousin, who has only one sickly child, the only heir of a large, undeserved fortune.

While most French authors agreed that the State should adopt measures to strengthen national character and urged populationist policies to remedy the *grève des ventres* (the strike of wombs),[73] interpretations of the fall of French natality varied a great deal. Some alleged the cause to be the weak fecundity of the race, while others invoked economic causes, such as the fragmentation of small property (a phenomenon in evidence since the Revolution), heavy taxation and the increased demand for leisure. Some said that the development of industry and trade had disproved Malthus's dire forecasts. Others thought it confirmed Malthus's doctrine of prudential restraint. Some took it as a confirmation of Spencer's law.[74] Others, like the Italian anthropologist Giuseppe Sergi[75] warned that it was a purely biological phenomenon of racial senescence wich had nothing to do with Malthus's principle. Race theorists like Georges Vacher de Lapouge[76] attributed it to the cross-breeding of the aristocratic 'dolicocephals' of Aryan origin with plebeian types.

The blame could be put on civilization itself. Far from being self-corrective – as Spencer thought – civilization was a threat to the quality and quantity of population. The most influential writers on depopulation (Le Play, Bertillon, Leroy-Beaulieu) sought a psychological, moral and social explanation of the phenomenon. Modern civilization, that is democracy, the economist Leroy-Beaulieu wrote, means 'the quasi-universal propagation of comfort and instruction, the soaring of individual and family ambition, the prospect open to all of elevating themselves in the social scale', but it also entails ambition, pursuit of pleasure, egoism, careerism, love of luxury, feminism, neo-Malthusianism ('the crime of Onan', as Bertillon put it).[77] In these circumstances children become a hindrance.

Arsène Dumont coined a successful term, 'social capillarity', to describe the process by which the individuals, like oil in the wick of a lamp, inevitably mount to higher levels in their social environment. In this upward movement they are interested mostly in doing what will benefit them personally, regardless of whether their behaviour will be of benefit to the community or race. As a consequence, they become less and less likely to reproduce themselves, because children impede the ascent. By the law of capillarity, 'which is to the social order what gravity is to the physical world', 'the development of numbers in a nation is in inverse ratio to the development of the individual'.[78] Social capillarity is greater where obstacles to movement from class to class are few. In France, where individualistic democracy is the well established fruit of the Revolution, mobility is great, and the birth rate suffers accordingly. In countries like India, where capillarity is checked by a rigid caste system, there is no tendency for population to decline. The same would hold true of the socialist society, where mobility would have no *raison d'être*. Socialize opportunity, equalize living conditions, and natality will rise.

As we shall soon see, this line of argument could easily shade into an attack on modernity and democracy, that is on civilization as such. Civilization, which had previously been invoked to dispel the spectre of overpopulation[79], was now accused of having done its job only too well.

Standard of living theories

Theories like Dumont's bear interesting similarities to those some German economists were elaborating at approximately the same time but in a different national context. Germany did experience a falling birth rate, but, in contrast to France, its population grew by 70% between 1866 and 1914. Malthusian economists such as Wagner, von Mohl, Schmoller, Roscher and Rümelin had attributed unemployment, pauperism, criminality, falling wages and all the evils from which the country suffered to overpopulation, and invoked State-enforced restrictions on marriages (as their colleagues had done successfully earlier in the century)[80].

Malthus's doctrine influenced the reform of the English Poor Laws (1834) and the restrictive marriage legislation in many German states, Austria and some Swiss cantons adopted in the 1820s. Unlike their British colleagues, the German Malthusians opted decisively for State-regulated marriage policies. This application of Malthus's teaching involved a deviation from the rules of conduct he prescribed, that is postponement of marriage and moral behaviour. But this deviation seemed to be justified by three factors: tremendous poverty, the unwillingness of gilds and wealthy citizens to allow freedom of movement (which seemed conducive to the rise of a landless proletariat) and the fear of revolution.[81] The connection between overpopulation and revolution was made quite clear by some of the participants in the debate: as the Bavarian minister Prince von Oettingen Wallenstein declared, 'it is necessary, by rendering marriage more difficult for the property-less, to bar the way to revolution'.[82] Some of the measures invoked brought ridicule and censure on their proponents as well as on Malthus himself. Others were so cruel as to provoke strong reactions even by some conservative thinkers.[83]

In Germany as elsewhere, as the threat of overpopulation seemed to fade away, some scholars challenged the Malthusian orthodoxy of political economists. Paul Mombert and Lujo Brentano, among others, contributed to the development of what came to be known as the 'standard of living theory' (*Wohlstandtheorie*). In environments of some physical comfort, they said, cultural factors (which they thought Malthus had underestimated) influence the people's choice between different forms of enjoyment available in that moment and at that stage of the evolution of society. Brentano, for instance, argued that sexual desire is no constant and regular motive as Malthus assumed, but is 'under the influence of mental activity'. The principal cause of the decline in fertility is the diminution of the desire for reproduction, as a consequence of the disinclination of the parents to being hampered in the enjoyment of other pleasures, or to being distracted from activities which render these other pleasures accessible. At a lower stage of civilization, and amongst the lower classes of the more advanced nations, there are no pleasures that enter into competition with the satisfaction derived from sexual intercourse. But as prosperity increases, so does the variety of pleasures which compete with marriage. It is economic causes that are especially responsible for the desire for reproduction: religion, race, occupation and all other factors are only relevant in so far as they affect material prosperity. Overpopulation is related to backwardness.[84]

This is a view which has become familiar to all of us. It is expressed in an argument over the relative merits of life back home and in Manhattan between two Puerto Rican girls in *West Side Story* (1957). Rosalia is homesick and dreams of the day when she will go back to her home village, whilst Anita is only too happy to have escaped from poverty and likes to be in America. She mocks her friend thus:

Anita: Puerto Rico...
You ugly island...
Island of tropic diseases.
Always the hurricanes blowing,
Always the population growing...
And the money owing,
And the babies crying,
And the bullets flying.

Rosalia: I like the city of San Juan ...
Hundreds of flowers in full bloom.

Anita: Hundreds of people in each room!

Survival of the unfittest

Brentano's theory was criticised even in Germany. Adolph Wagner defined it 'a hypothesis as arbitrary as the mystical laws of Spencer and Carey'. Julius Wolf accused Brentano of neglecting the decisive importance of world views and values (as manifested in religion, ideologies, sexual moral, feminism etc.) in determining behaviour. He argued for instance that the reduction of fertility in some regions of Germany and in some parts of the population was in fact due to the influence of Catholicism. Mombert and Brentano replied that the influence of ideological factors varied according to the economic and social level of the people concerned, in a word according to the degree of civilization they had reached: Catholics, for instance, behaved differently in industrial or rural districts.[85] Other commentators remarked that, in its original formulation, the standard-of-living theory did not take into account a fact whose dramatic importance had been increasingly recognized in recent years. 'It is a phenomenon very generally observed', wrote the American sociologist Warren S. Thompson, 'that where peoples of different standards of living, whose cultures are not too widely different, come into contact, those having lower standards of living supplant those having higher standards'.[86] This caused a struggle for the means of subsistence not much different from that described by Malthus: only, 'the process of starvation is more refined' today.[87] Therefore, Thompson went on to say, if we want to mitigate the pressure upon the means of subsistence and the suffering due to overcrowding, 'either our present standard of living must be simplified as an increasing proportion of the population becomes rural or the present rate of increase of population must be lowered. Probably both must take place in order to have a really progressive civilization'. A greater control over the growth of population 'will give more time to adjust standards of life to surrounding conditions and to direct the course of progress'.[88] But 'if population must increase more slowly, from what part of the population should this increase come?' Rational social control entails 'a study of the eugenic value of the different classes of the population'.[89] Progress requires social selection.

Brentano's theory, too, was based on a belief in progress. But he saw no reason to fear that European civilization was threatened. Many of his contemporaries, however, were much less sanguine. To them, the global decline of the national population was only one side of the problem. The other was something Malthus could not even imagine: its increasingly poor quality, due to changes in the relative numbers of its better and its worse elements. While the better classes, being more prudent, restricted their offspring, low-quality proletarians multiplied recklessly and threatened to outbreed them. Under these conditions, as Galton and Greg warned as early as the 1860s, the prudential check invoked by Malthus would operate against the interests of the race. Differential fertility was more alarming than present general decline and past overpopulation. As the historian Richard Soloway[90] has put it, the danger of the survival of the unfittest 'was a danger of relative, not absolute depopulation'. Not mere lack of prudence but biological taint was the disease; not vice and misery, but degeneration of the whole race its consequence. The Darwinian world now rebelled against its Malthusian father.

In these circumstances, both Malthusian and Spencerian attitudes shared the same fate. If Malthus' recommendations could be detrimental, and if no law of a Spencerian kind could come to the rescue (as in Greg's and Bagehot's case), then nature's laws needed man's help. The situation called for eugenic measures, which were discussed with different emphases in different countries.[91] In Britain and in the United States eugenic thinking was based predominantly on selectionist principles: the nation stock had to be improved by multiplying its best members, that is by raising the fertility of the higher and the middle classes.[92] An increasing stress on State intervention led to a decline of traditional *laissez-faire*. State intervention was much more strongly invoked by adherents of the German *Rassenhygiene*, many of whom approved of some form of State socialism (which they eventually found in Nazism); German race hygienists stressed the duty of the individual to the race and his subordination to the community.[93] In France, the prevailing Lamarckian mood and the emphasis on the Third Republic ideology of solidarity led to campaigning for education, radical reform and public health, in the hope that a better quality of life would improve the biological quality of the population.[94]

There were many varieties of eugenics, and no common attitude of eugenicists towards Malthus and the neo-Malthusians, who argued that until the increase of population was substantially curtailed, poverty would remain endemic and economic growth would be constrained. Some supported birth control; others thought Malthus was basically right, but neo-Malthusian propaganda should not be spread indiscriminately. Still others denounced the desire to limit the number of children as 'an imminent danger to the country, and high treason to the human race',[95] or deplored birth control as having dysgenic effects and giving 'aid to luxury and convenience'[96]. Birth control, argued the German racial hygienist Alfred Ploetz, led to the degeneration of the race.[97] Sterilization of the undesirable was preferable. Contraception was rejected even by those who invoked forced sterilization. As late as 1939, a Nazi doctor said that Malthus and his followers had 'declared war on the child', and that the Nazis must struggle against the 'Malthusian' poison (by which he meant contraception and birth control).[98] In 1932 the leading eugenicist Eugen Fischer described the condition of the German people as that of a 'dying people': an unprecedented population catastrophe had occurred, bringing the average number of children per family down from 3.37 (between 1879 and 1886) to 2.65 (between 1907 and 1910), with university professors having now 2.8 children and peasants 6.5.[99]

Kulturpessimismus

Although eugenicists vacillated between anxiety and confidence, their activism stood in striking contrast with the fatalistic pessimism which increasingly characterized other critics of Western society, especially in Germany. These critics used against modern civilization as a whole many of the arguments that had long been employed against urbanization, industrialization, enlightenment and democracy. Concern for population became part of the concern for the fate of the whole of Western civilization. Population movements formed part of the behavioural characteristics typical of each phase of the life-cycle of nations (or races, or civilizations), that is of universal processes beyond rational control. Stages and cycles of population corresponded to the stages and cycles of civilization. As nations passed through an evolutionary parabola, ending their predestined course in decline and death, so did racial reproductive vigour fatally rise and fall.[100] The greatest cultural flowering was accompanied by the seeds of inevitable downfall. Like effeminate manners, luxury, urban growth, decadent art and so forth, decline in fertility was perceived as an indication of imminent decay. In this, the *Kulturpessimisten* joined hands with some representatives of that very positivistic science they despised. For many medical and biological authorities had associated sterility and degeneration.[101]

In works like Oswald Spengler's greatly successful *Decline of the West* (1918-1922) culture ceased to be a set of interrelated factors, each having its differential influence on sexual behaviour. It became the manifestation of an almighty force which pervaded all aspects of life. It was an agent of doom subjugating the individual to a destiny on which he had no control. Spengler included sexual mores in his attack on modernity. Moral restraint was a symptom of the deadly disease which would bring the West to its grave, and which consisted in the predominance of reasoning, calculation and effete refinement over instinct, spontaneous creativity and immediate contact with the obscure forces of life. The strength of a race, he said in a later work published in the same year in which the Nazis seized power, is seen in its 'spontaneous natural fertility', and in its power to repair losses. But the peoples of white race were drained of energies. Their will to power and vital instincts were exhausted. The irresistible craving for immortality, glory, and conquest which characterizes healthy nations and manifests itself in a numerous family was lost. 'The vulgar doctrine of Malthus that prizes sterility as a progress' was itself a sign of decadence: the very fact that the number of children had become a matter of rational choice demonstrated that instinct had dwindled. The 'suicide of the white race' opened the way for the 'world revolution of the coloured races'. Salvation was possible only for the race in whose blood there had survived 'a spark of primeval barbarity', that is of 'the eternal warlike element typical of Man the beast of prey'. Needless to say, the German were the people who had least wasted their vital energy. But they should be prepared to endure 'a stern selection by hardship of life, diseases and war'. The 'decisive years' after the catastrophe of 1918 were no time for adding the 'moral disarmament of pacifism' to the 'physical disarmament of sterility'.[102] In Spengler's view of the human predicament, social factors as such had disappeared. Historical factors were absorbed into the unfathomable category of destiny. Biological factors were replaced by a misty mythology of blood and fate.

It may seem arbitrary to conclude this *tour d'horizon* here. But it is not entirely so. It is as though those who appealed to nature against the Malthusian threat had summoned forces that were now used against them. Spengler's case shows how dangerous it is in ideological controversies to appeal to entities that transcend human reason, whether they be Nature, Life, Providence, History or Evolution. Optimistic believers in the beneficent order of things thought they had nature on their side in their struggle against the dismal parson. Spengler went further, and fielded an even more powerful ally: Destiny. But he used it against both those who thought that population problems could be tackled by applying reason and those who invoked some form of higher rationality embodied in providence or evolution. Malthusians, socialists, Darwinians, positivist sociologists, economists were all alike tainted with the original sin of Western modernity: rationality. The issue of population was now, so to speak, dispersed in a cosmical *mise en question* of civilization itself. Nothing less than a world catastrophe could act as a positive check to the proliferation of such an idea.

Acknowledgement

I am very grateful to Daniel Pick for commenting on an earlier draft of this paper, and to Brian Dolan for his editorial work.

Biology and Sociology of Fertility

Notes

1. Samuel M. Levin, 'Malthus and the Idea of Progress', *Journal of the History of Ideas*, 27 (1966), 92-108; D.L. LeMahieu, 'Malthus and the theodicy of scarcity', *Journal of the History of Ideas*, 40 (1979), 467-474; J.M. Pullen, 'Malthus' theological ideas and their influence on his principle of population', *History of Political Economy*, 13 (1981), 39-54; E.N. Santurri, 'Theodicy and social policy in Malthus' thought', *Journal of the History of Ideas*, 63 (1982), 315-330; D. Wells, 'Resurrecting the dismal parson: Malthus, ecology and political thought', *Political Studies*, 30 (1982), 1-15; A.M.C. Waterman, 'Malthus as a theologian: the *First Essay* and the relation between political economy and Christian theology', in J. Dupâquier, A. Fauve-Chamoux, and E. Grebenik (eds), *Malthus Past and Present* (London and New York: Academic Press, 1983), 195-209; Antonello La Vergata, *Nonostante Malthus. Fecondità, popolazioni e armonia della natura, 1700-1900* (Torino: Bollati Boringhieri, 1990), chapter 3.
2. See La Vergata, *Nonostante Malthus*, chapter 4, where works by John Weyland, Michael Thomas Sadler and Thomas Doubleday are discussed in detail.
3. Carey invoked cosmical harmony to support his theories both before and after abandoning *laissez-faire* for protectionism. Apparently, the argument from harmony could serve all purposes.
4. See the discussion of Petty, Graunt, Süssmilch and other early demographers in La Vergata, *Nonostante Malthus*, chapter 2.
5. For instance, the historian and Tory Sheriff of Lanarckshire, Sir Archibald Alison, *The Principles of Population, and Their Connection with Human Happiness* (Edinburgh, W. Blackwood & Sons, 1840), I, 107-111, stressed the importance of social emulation and of 'the extension of artificial wants', especially among the inhabitants of towns, as factors that limit population growth. He argued that prudence increases in proportion to ranks, and he mentioned as evidence 'the common observation, that the nobility of every country are on the decline'. The Genevan economist Simonde de Sismondi, *Nouveaux principes d'économie politique, ou, De la richesse dans ses rapports avec la population* (original 1819; Paris, Delaunay, 1827), II, 252, stated clearly that 'the multiplication of the [human] species depends on the will, and it is in this will that it has its limits'. No positive check, he added, prevented noble and rich families like the Montmorency from increasing their numbers, but by 1800 they were virtually extinct.
6. See for instance Julien-Joseph Virey, 'Fécondité', *Dictionnaire des*

211

sciences médicales, par une société de médecins et de chirurgiens (Paris, Panckoucke, 1815), XIV, 480–97.

7. For instance Richard Price, *Observations on reversionary payments...*, second edition, with a supplement (London, Cadell, 1772), 354, 359–62; Price, *An essay on the population of England, from the revolution to the present time* (London, Cadell, 1780), 63.

8. Alfred Marshall, *Principles of Economics. An introductory volume*, 8th ed. (London, Macmillan, 1920 (orig. 1890)), 185; Frank H. Hankins, 'Does Advancing Civilization involve a Decline in Natural Fertility?', *Studies in Quantitative and Cultural Sociology. Papers Presented at the Twenty-forth Annual Meeting of the American Sociological Society, held at Washington, D.C., December 27-30, 1929, Publications of the American Sociological Society*, (Chicago: University of Chicago Press, 1930), XIV, 115–22; *idem*, 'Has the Reproductive Power of Western Peoples Declined?', in G.H.L.F. Pitt-Rivers (ed.), *Problems of Population. Being the Report of the Proceedings of the Second General Assembly of the International Union for the Scientific Investigation of Population Problems, held at the Royal Society of Arts*, London, June 15–18, 1931 (London: George Allen & Unwin, 1932; reprinted. Port Washington, New York and London: Kennikat Press, 1971), 181–8. Marshall believed that fertility was reduced by both physiological and psychological factors (depending on cultural and social level). Hankins endorsed an updated version of Spencer's theory discussed below.

9. Instances are given in La Vergata, *Nonostante Malthus*, chapter 4.

10. Thomas Short, *New observations, natural, moral, civil, poltical and medical on city, town, and country bills of mortality*, (1750) reprinted with an introduction by R. Wall (Farnborough, Hants.: Gregg, 1973), 144.

11. Short, *New Observations*, 145: 'For here we see a Chain of Providences and Blessings attends the Virtue, Industry, Chastity, Sobriety, Regularity, poor, but plain Food of poor labouring People; they are less Slaves to the sensual passion, are more fruitful, their Progeny more vigorous and healthy, have fewer hereditary Diseases, and sooner and more easily overcome the common ones, have stronger Constitutions, and better Stamina, relish a more natural and true Pleasure in Wedlock...'

12. Price, *Observations on Reversionary Payments*, 354.

13. R. Freedman, 'Fertility', in D.L. Sills (ed.), *International Encyclopaedia of the Social Sciences* (Washington: The Macmillan Company and The Free Press /Crowell Collier and Macmillan, 1968), V, 371–82.

14. James Matthew Duncan, *Fecundity, Fertility, Sterility and Allied Topics* (1866), second edition, revised and enlarged (Edinburgh, Adam and Charles Black, 1871), 3.

15. So does, for instance, Hankins (see his 'Does Advancing Civilization involve a Decline in Natural Fertility?' and 'Has the Reproductive Power of Western Peoples Declined?') who uses 'natural fertility', 'innate fecundity' and other terms as equivalent, and at times as synonymous with 'sexual vigour' at large.

16. W. Petersen, *Malthus* (London: Heinemann, 1979), 64.

17. See for instance Ruth Schwarz Cowan, 'Nature and nurture. The interplay of biology and politics in the work of Francis Galton' *Studies in the History of Biology* 1 (1977), 133–207, and the works mentioned in note 91.

18. Robert M. Young, 'The historiographic and ideological contexts of the nineteenth century debate on man's place in nature', in M. Teich and R.M. Young (eds), *Changing Perspectives in the History of Science* (London: Heinemann, 1973), 344–438.

19. William E. Hickson, *Malthus. An Essay on the Principle of Population in Refutation of the Rev. T. R. Malthus* (London: Taylor, Walton and Maberley, 1849), 183; originally in *Westminster Review* 52 (1849–1850), 133–201.

20. Thomas Jarrold, *Dissertations on Man, Philosophical, Physiological, and Political; in Answer to Mr. Malthus' 'Essay on the Principle of Population'* (London: Caddell and Davis, 1806).

21. Michael Thomas Sadler, *The Law of Population: a Treatise, in Six Books; in Disproof of the Superfecundity of Human Beings, and Developing the Real Principle of their Increase* (London: Murray, 1830).

22. Charles Loudon, *The Equilibrium of Population and Sustenance Demonstrated; Showing on Physiological and Statistical Grounds the Means of Obviating the Fears of the Late Mr. Malthus and His Followers* (Leamington Spa, printed by James Fairfax and sold by Longman, Rees, Orme & Co., London, 1836).

23. George (Simon Gray) Purves, *Gray vs. Malthus. The principles of population and production investigated; and the question: Does population regulate subsistence, or subsistence population... etc. discussed* (London: Longman, Hurst, Rees, Orme and Brown, 1818); Thomas Doubleday, *The True law of Population, Shewn to be Connected with the Food of People* (London: George Peirce, 1842).

24. Virey, 'Fécondité', 485–486. As late as the end of the nineteenth century many doctors believed that spasms without insemination damaged the female body: this opinion was held, for instance, by

(Jean-Louis-François-Etienne Bergeret, *Des fraudes dans l'accomplissement des fonctions génératrices; causes, dangers et inconvénients pour les individus, la famille et la société* (Paris: Baillière, 1868)) and other medical authorities consulted by Emile Zola when writing his novel *Fécondité* (1899).

25. Herbert Spencer, 'A Theory of Population, Deduced from the General Law of Animal Fertility' *Westminster Review* 57 (o.s.), 16 (n.s.) (1852), 468–501, pp. 492–3.

26. *Ibid.*, 501, 506. I have discussed the context of this doctrine of Spencer's in La Vergata, *Nonostante Malthus*, chapter 5.

27. Gide dropped support to Spencer's law from later edition of his book, written with the collaboration of Charles Rist, *Principes d'Economie politique* (Paris, 1883; reprint Paris, Libraire du Recueil Sirey, 1920). Vilfredo Pareto, *Cours d'économie politique* (Lausanne: Rouge, 1896), I, § 192, wrote that Spencer's law could be true, but its effects were too slow. Pareto considered Malthus's theory 'a theory with a true foundation, now well now deplorably argued, from which erroneous consequences are drawn' (117). Spencer's article was reprinted without mentioning Spencer's name in America by a well-known physician and hydropath, Dr. Russell Thacher Trall (*A new theory of population, republished from the 'Westminster Review', for April, 1852, with an introduction by R. T. Trall* (New York: Fowler and Wells, 1857), and then translated into German as Trall's own work (1877). Carey (*Principles of Social Science*, Philadelphia: Lippincott & Co., 1858–59; reprinted New York: Augustus M. Kelley, Librarian, 1963) read the original and used it to support his philosophy of universal harmony. Indeed, his theory of the antagonism between the nervous and sexual functions bears such striking similarities with that of Spencer that one is tempted to think he copied from him altogether.

28. William Rathbone Greg, 'Malthus Notwithstanding', in *Enigmas of Life* (original 1872), ninth edition, with a postscript (London: N. Trübner & Co., 1874), 75, italics in original.

29. *Ibid.*, 42.

30. *Ibid.*, 124.

31. William Rathbone Greg, 'On the Failure of Natural Selection in the Case of Man' *Fraser's Magazine* 78 (1868), 353–362, p. 361.

32. Walter Bagehot, 'Economic Studies: Malthus' (1880), in Norman St. John-Stevas (ed.), *The Collected Works of Walter Bagehot* (London: The Economist, 1978), XI, 336.

33. Patrick Geddes and John Arthur Thomson, *The Evolution of Sex* (London: W. Scott, 1889), 292.

34. *Ibid.*
35. Wladimir Berelovitch, 'Les lectures de Malthus en Russie', in Antoinette Fauve-Chamoux (ed.), *Malthus hier et aujourd'hui* (Paris: Editions du CNRS, 1984), 405–15; Daniel P. Todes, *Darwin Without Malthus: the Struggle for Existence in Russian Evolutionary Thought* (Oxford: Oxford University Press, 1989).
36. This was Godwin's idea, and one cherished by many reformers, not only socialists. Hickson (*Malthus*, 73) for instance, believed hat a better organization of production and distribution in future society would lead to great changes in the very nature of man: 'the strength of mere animal propensies would diminish, and [...] in accordance with the law that the highest organizations should be the most slowly developed, the ratio of increase would be less than at present'. Malthus (*An Essay on the Principle of Population, and A Summary View of the Principle of Population*, edited by A. Flew (Harmondsworth: Penguin Books, 1976), 114) had aswered Godwin by saying that attraction between the sexes 'has appeared in every age to be so nearly the same that it may alwys be considered, in algebraic language, as a given quantity'.
37. François-Marie-Charles Fourier, *Le nouveau monde industriel et sociétaire, ou invention des procédés d'industrie attrayante et naturelle distribuée en séries passionnées*, originally published 1829–30 (Bruxelles: A la Librairie belge-française, 1840), II, 158–63.
38. Pierre-Joseph Proudhon, *Système des contradictions économiques, ou philosophie de la misère* (Paris: Guillaumin, 1846), II, 477–8.
39. Proudhon, *De la justice dans la révolution et dans l'église* (Paris: Garnier Frères, 1858), I, 327–34, 347.
40. Engels, *Umrisse einer Kritik der Nationalökonomie* (1844), cit. by Ludwig Elster, 'Bevölkerungswesen (Bevölkerungslehre und Bevölkerungspolitik)', in *Handwörterbuch der Staatswissenschaften*, hrsg. von L. Elster, A Weber und F. Wieser, vierte gänzlich umgearbeitete Auflage, 2. Band (Jena: Fischer, 1924), 774.
41. Karl Marx, *Capital. A Critical Analysis of Capitalist Production*, transl. from the 3rd German edited by Samuel Moore and Edward Aveling, and edited by F. Engels (London: William Glaisher, 1918), 645.
42. *Ibid.*
43. *Ibid.*, 658.
44. *Ibid.*, 627.
45. *Ibid.*, 648.
46. *Ibid.*, 657.
47. As Robert M. Young remarked in his 'Malthus and the evolutionists: the common context of biological and social theory' *Past and Present*

43 (1969), 109–145. On Marx's and Engels' attacks on Malthus see Samuel M. Levin, 'Marx *vs.* Malthus' *Michigan Academy of Science, Arts and Letters* 22 (1936), 243–58; R.L. Meek, *Marx and Engels on Malthus* (London: Lawrence and Wishart, 1953).

48. Karl Kautsky, *Der Einfluss der Volksvermehrung auf den Fortschritt der Gesellschaft* (Wien: Bloch und Hasbach, 1880).

49. On Italian debates over Malthus and population see Teresa Isemburg, 'Il dibattito su Malthus e sulla popolazione nell'Italia di fine '800', *Studi storici* 18 (1977), 41–67; Luigi Pucci, '"Popolazione eccedente" e industrialismo. Alcune osservazioni sulla controversia malthusiana in Italia nel XIX secolo', *Cahiers internationaux d'histoire économique et sociale* 12 (1980), 115–40; Claudio Pogliano, 'L'enigma demologico. Natalità, popolazione, socialismo (1880–1900)', *Schema* 7 (1985), 1–42; Carl Ipsen, *Dictating Demography. The Problem of Population in Fascist Italy* (Berkeley: University of California Press, 1992).

50. S.M. Ganci (ed.), *Democrazia e socialismo in Italia. Il carteggio di Napoleone Colajanni, 1878-1898* (Milano: Feltrinelli, 1959), 125.

51. Leonida Bissolati, *Contadini del Circondario di Cremona* (Cremona: Tipografia Sociale, 1886), 56, quoted approvingly by Colajanni, 'Fatti e teorie', *Rivista italiana del socialismo*, 1 (1886), 40–43, 43.

52. One of the chapters of Colajanni (*Il socialismo* (1884), 2nd edn (Palermo and Milano: Sandron, 1898)) was entitled 'Spencer's ideal is a socialistic one'. Needless to say, Spencer protested, and in the second edition of the book (1898), Colajanni suppressed the chapter. In the preface, he justified himself by saying that in 1884 he did not know that Spencer had reneged the ideas put forth in *Social statics* (1851). See also Colajanni, 'Per una lettera di Spencer', *Rivista repubblicana di politica, filosofia, scienze e letteratura*, 15 July 1895. Strange though it may seem, Colajanni's misunderstanding was a very common one, not only in Italy. The tendency to reconcile Spencer's cosmical evolutionism with socialism reached its apex in Enrico Ferri, *Socialismo e scienza positiva (Darwin, Spencer, Marx)* (Roma: Casa Editrice Sociale, 1894), which enjoyed great success and was translated into many languages.

53. Colajanni, *Il socialismo*, 109, 112, 114–5.

54. Filippo Turati, 'Malthusianismo vecchio e nuovo' (review of Kautsky 1884), *Il Secolo* (Milan), 19 (16–17 June 1884).

55. Turati, 'La propaganda fra i contadini e la legge di Malthus', *Critica sociale* 2 (1892), 236.

56. Turati, 'Fra un libro e l'altro', *La farfalla*, 7 October 1883, quoted in Pogliano, 'L'enigma demologico', 16. Cf. Turati, 'La propaganda fra i

contadini e la legge di Malthus', *Critica sociale* 2 (1892), 236.

57. Joseph J. Spengler, 'French Population Theory since 1800', *Journal of Political Economy* 44 (1936), 577–611, 743–66, 753.

58. Leonida Bissolati, 'Il socialismo e il problema della popolazione', *Critica sociale* 2 (1892), 245–247, 246.

59. In Italy as in other countries attitudes towards Malthus were influenced by the diffusion of neo-Malthusianism (the two being often confused). An Italian translation of Drysdale's neo-Malthusian treatise *Elements of Social Science, or Physical, Sexual and Natural Religion* was published in 1874.

60. Francesco Saverio Nitti, *Population and the Social System*, translated under the author's supervision (London: Swan Sonnenschein, 1894), 167 (originally published as *La popolazione e il sistema sociale*, Turin, Le Roux, 1894).

61. Nitti, *Population and the Social System*, 188. The English translation says 'anatomical and physical', but the Italian original (198) has 'psichici'.

62. Nitti, *Population and the Social System*, 171.

63. Karl Kautsky, *Vermehrung und Entwicklung in Natur und Gesellschaft* (Stuttgart: Dietz, 1910), 25.

64. *Ibid.*, 33.

65. *Ibid.*, 252.

66. C.V. Drysdale, eugenicist, quoted in W. Petersen, *Malthus* (London: Heinemann, 1979), 198.

67. Dr Oguse, cit. in Francis Ronsin, *La grève des ventres. Propagande néo-malthusienne et baisse de la natalité en France (XIXe-XXe siècles)* (Paris: Aubier Montaigne, 1980), 175.

68. On the attitude of socialists towards population problems and birth control see André Armengaud, 'Mouvement ouvrier et néo-malthusianisme au début du XXe siècle', *Annales de démographie historique* 3 (1966), 7–21; Léon Gani, 'Jules Guesde, Paul Lafargue et les problèmes de la population', *Population* 34 (1979), 1023–1043; the essays in Dupâquier, Fauve-Chamoux, and Grebenik (eds), *Malthus Past and Present*; Diane Paul, 'Eugenics and the Left', *Journal of the History of Ideas* 45 (1984), 567–90; Marcel Schneider, 'The eugenics movement in France, 1890-1945', in Mark B. Adams (ed.), *The Wellborn Science. Eugenics in Germany, France, Brazil, and Russia* (New York and Oxford: Oxford University Press, 1990), 69–109, and the works cited in Angus McLaren, *Sexuality and the social order. The debate over the fertility of women and workers in France, 1770-1920* (New York: Holmes and Meier, 1983), 303–304, notes 73–6.

69. Richard A. Soloway, *Demography and Degeneration: Eugenics and the Declining Birthrate in Twentieth-Century Britain* (Chapel Hill: University of North Carolina Press, 1990), 4.

70. Spengler, 'French Population Theory since 1800'; Spengler, *France Faces Depopulation* (Durham, NC: Duke University Press, 1938); Yves Charbit, *Du malthusianisme au populationnisme. Les économistes français et la population, 1840-1870*, préface d'Alfred Sauvy (Paris: Presses Universitaires de France, 1981); McLaren, *Sexuality and the social order.*

71. Jean-Marie Guyau, *L'irreligion de l'avenir. Etude sociologique* (Paris: Alcan, 1887), 281, 276.

72. 'O mères françaises, faites donc des enfants, pour que la France garde son rang, sa force et sa prosperité, car il est nécessaire au salut du monde que la France vive, elle d'où est partie l'émancipation humaine, elle d'où partiront toute vérité et toute justice! Si elle doit un jour ne faire plus qu'un avec l'humanité, ce sera comme la mer où tous les fleuves viennent se perdre. Et je voudrais, chez elle, que le déchet de la vie cessât, que la vie fût adorée comme la bonne déesse, l'immortelle, celle qui donne l'éternelle victoire' (Zola, *Nouvelle campagne, 1896* (Paris: Charpentier, 1897), quoted in Armengaud, *Les Français et Malthus* (Paris: Press Universitaires de France, 1975), 104.

73. This is the title of a book by the neo-Malthusian Fernand Kolney (Paris: Edition de 'Génération consciente', 1908).

74. Gaétan Delaunay, 'La fécondité', *Revue scientifique* (Revue rose), 22.me année, troisième série, t. X (1885), 434–6, 466–70.

75. Giuseppe Sergi and Filippo Turati, 'Due obiezioni alle nostre idee sulla legge di Malthus e sul valore sociale della donna', *Critica sociale* 3 (1893), 245–9.

76. Georges Vacher de Lapouge, *Les sélections sociales* (Paris: Fontemoing, 1896).

77. Paul Leroy-Beaulieu, *La question de la population*, deuxième édition revue et corrigée (Paris: Alcan, 1913). Cf. Jacques Bertillon, *La dépopulation de la France. Ses causes. Mesures à prendre pour la combattre* (Paris: Alcan, 1911), 101.

78. Arsène Dumont, *La Morale basée sur la démographie* (Paris: Schleicher frères, 1901), 33.

79. See for instance E.A. Ross, 'Civilization and birth rate', *American Journal of Sociology*, 12 (1906-1907), 607–17.

80. Elster, 'Bevölkerungswesen (Bevölkerungslehre und Bevölkerungspolitik)'.

81. Rolf Peter Sieferle, *Bevölkerungswachstum und Naturhaushalt. Studien zur Naturtheorie der klassischen Ökonomie* (Frankfurt: Suhrkamp

Verlag, 1990).

82. Quoted in Elster, 'Bevölkerungswesen (Bevölkerungslehre und Bevölkerungspolitik)', 771.
83. See for instance Franz von Baader's attack ('Reflexion über einen neulich öffentlich gemacht scandalösen Vorschlag gegen Überbevölkerung', *Eos* 12 (1828), 698–9) on Weinhold's proposal (*Von der Übervölkerung in Mittel-Europa und deren Folgen auf die Staaten und deren Civilisation* (Halle 1827)) of mass male infibulation. In a pamphlet published in England in 1830 under the pseudonym of Marcus (*On the possibility of limiting pompousness*, reprinted in W. Dugdale, *The book of murder. Vademecum for the commissioners and guardians of the New Poor Law throughout Great Britain and Ireland, being an exact reprint of the infamous essay: On the possibility of limiting populousness, by Marcus with a refutation of the Malthusian doctrine*, (London: J. Hill, 1839)) it was argued that the State should organize a public service to put excess poor children to death painlessly (for instance by gas-poisoning them). It was probably a provocation in a time of Chartist agitation (Harold Boner, *Hungry Generations. The Nineteenth-century Case against Malthusianism* (New York: King's Crown Press, 1955), but some people, including Engels, took it seriously: he thought the book brought Malthus' ideas to their extreme but logical consequences.
84. Lujo Brentano, 'Die Malthussche Lehre und die Bevölkerungsbewegung der letzten Dezennien', *Abhandlungen der historischen Klasse der Königlich Bayerischen Akademie der Wissenschaften* XXIV Bd., III Abt. (1909), 567–625 (Anhang); Lujo Brentano, 'The Doctrine of Malthus and the Increase of Population During the Last Decades', *Economic Journal* 20 (1910), 371–93. In England Arthur Newsholme and Stevenson ('The decline of human fertility in the United Kingdom and other countries as shown by correlated birth rates', *Journal of the Royal Statistical Society* 69 (1906), 34–87) had reached the same conclusion: '[The decline of human fertility] is associated with a general raising of the standard of comfort; and is an expression of the determination of the people to secure this greater comfort. It is not caused by a greater stress in modern life, but is a consequence of a greater desire for luxury'. Neither increased nutrition nor increased mental and moral development were important factors in the decline of the birth rate. Nutrition could be responsible in part, but, if so, not because it produced physiological alterations: it acted by influencing the state of mind and ultimately through the will.
85. Adolph Wagner, *Agrar- und Industriestaat. Die Kehrseite des*

Industriestaates und die Rechtfertigung agrarischen Zollschutzes, mit besonderer Rücksicht auf die Bevölkerungsfrage, zweite, grossenteils umgearbeitete und stark vermehrte Auflage (Jena: Fischer, 1902) (orig. 1901). But see Heinrich Dietzel, 'Die Streit um Malthus' Lehre', *Festgaben für Adolf Wagner zur siebzigsten Wiederkehr seines Geburtstages,* (Leipzig: Winter, 1905), 20–52, 42, who tries to reconcile his position with Brentano's; Julius Wolf, *Der Geburtenrückgang. Die Rationaliesierung der Sexuallebens in unserer Zeit* (Jena: Fischer, 1912). For a short discussion see Max Scheler, 'Bevölkerungsprobleme als Weltanschauungsfragen' (1921), in *Gesammelte Werke,* Bd. 6: *Schriften zur Soziologie und Weltanschauungslehre,* 2nd edn (Bern und München: Francke Verlag, 1963), 290–324, pp. 297–99.

86. Warren S. Thompson, *Population: a Study in Malthusianism* (New York: Columbia University, 1915), 159.

87. *Ibid.,* 163.

88. *Ibid.,* 164.

89. *Ibid.,* 165.

90. Soloway, *Demography and Degeneration.*

91. Secondary literature on eugenics is constantly increasing: see Geoffrey Searle, *Eugenics and politics in Britain, 1900-1914* (Leyden: Brill, 1976); Paul Weindling, *Health, Race and German Politics between National Unification and Nazism, 1870-1945* (Cambridge: Cambridge University Press, 1989); Mark B. Adams (ed.), *The Wellborn Science. Eugenics in Germany, France, Brazil, and Russia* (New York and Oxford: Oxford University Press, 1990); Angus McLaren, *Our own master race. Eugenics in Canada* (Toronto: McClelland and Stewart, 1990); Pauline Mazumdar, *Eugenics, human genetics and human failings. The Eugenics Society, its sources and its critics in Britain* (London: Routledge, 1992); and Daniel J. Kevles, *In the Name of Eugenics: Genetics and the Uses of Human Heredity* (Cambridge, MA: Harvard University Press, 1995 (orig. 1985)). On the fear of degeneration see Daniel Pick, *Faces of Degeneration. A European Disorder, 1848-1918* (Cambridge: Cambridge University Press, 1989).

92. Concern for eugenics stimulated much statistical work. For instance, it was under the auspices of Karl Pearson's Eugenics Laboratory, and as the first contribution to a series of studies in national deterioration, that a detailed research on differential fertility and mortality, the statistician's David Heron's *On the relation of fertility in man to social status and the changes in this relation that have taken place during the last fifty years,* was published in 1906.

93. Sheila Faith Weiss, *Race Hygiene and National Efficiency: the Eugenics of*

Wilhelm Schallmayer (Berkeley: University of California Press, 1987).

94. Marcel Schneider, 'The eugenics movement in France, 1890-1945', in Adams (ed.), *The Wellborn Science*, 69–109.

95. As the English physicist W.C.D. Whetham and his wife Catherine wrote in their book *The Family and the Nation* (1909) (cit. in Kevles, *In the Name of Eugenics*, 73).

96. C. Davenport, American biologist, quoted in Kevles, *In the Name of Eugenics*, 53. The idea that contraception fostered licentiousness was shared by Darwin. He refused to be subpoenaed in the Bradlaugh and Besant trial of 1877 for obscenity: in a letter to Bradlaugh he said that artificial checks to the natural rate of human increase are undesirable, and the use of of artificial means to prevent conception would destroy chastity and ultimately the family (Hypatia Bradlaugh Bonner, *Charles Bradlaugh: a record of his life and work* (London: T. Fisher Unwin, 1894), 2: 24).

97. Alfred Ploetz, *Die Tüchtigkeit unsrer Rasse. Ein Versuch über Rassenhygiene und ihr Verhältnis zu den humanen Idealen, besonders zum Sozialismus* (Berlin: Fischer, 1895), 202–7.

98. Ludwig Schmidt-Kehl, quoted in Robert N. Proctor, *Racial Hygiene. Medicine under the Nazis* (Cambridge, MA: Harvard University Press, 1988), 342, 30f.

99. Eugen Fischer, 'Untersuchungen über die differenzierte Fortpflanzung am deutschen Volk nach Hermann Muckermann', in Pitt-Rivers (ed.), *Problems of Population*, 108–11.

100. Georg Hansen, *Die drei Bevölkerungsstufen. Ein Versuch, die Ursachen für das Blühen und Altern der Völker nachzuweisen* (München: Lindauer, 1889); P.E. Fahlbeck, 'La décadence et la chute des peuples', *Bulletin International de Statistique*, 15 (1900); Corrado Gini, *I fattori demografici dell'evoluzione delle nazioni* (Torino: Bocca, 1912); *idem*, 'The cyclical rise and fall of population', in Gini *et al.*, *Population. Lectures on the Harris Foundation, 1929* (Chicago: University of Chicago Press, 1930); *idem, Nascita, evoluzione e morte delle nazioni. La teoria ciclica della popolazione e i vari sistemi di politica demografica* (Roma: Libreria del Littorio, 1930); *idem, Teorie della popolazione* (Roma: Casa editrice Castellani, 1945). On Gini see Ipsen, *Dictating demography* and Roberto Maiocchi, *Scienza italiana e razzismo fascista* (Firenze: La Nuova Italia, 1999). Gini believed that the reproductive capability varied inversely not only with culture, but also with the age of a people: highly civilized nations have an old, less effective 'germ plasm'; this is why they are less aggressive than young ascending, though coarse, ones.

101. For instance, Charles Robin had declared in the 1860s: 'Final sterility

is a criterion of degeneration. Everything that is conducive to it is a stage of degeneration'. Conversely, degeneration was defined as a series of organic and functional alterations that can be transmitted by inheritance and result in sterility' (quoted in Claude Bénichou, 'Enquête et réflexions sur l'introduction des termes 'dégénéré(r), 'dégénération', 'dégénérescence' dans les dictionnaires et encyclopédies scientifiques françaises à partir du 17ème siècle', *Documents pour l'histoire du vocabulaire scientifique*, Paris: Publications de l'Institut de la langue française, 5 (1993), 1–83, 57.

102. Spengler, *Jahre der Entscheidung* (München: Beck, 1933), 157–62.

Index

223

PHILIP K. WILSON

Surgery, Skin and Syphilis:
Daniel Turner's London (1667-1741)

Amsterdam/Atlanta, GA 1999. XVI,312 pp.
(Clio Medica 54/The Wellcome Institute Series in the History
of Medicine)
ISBN: 90-420-0526-2   Bound Hfl. 160,-/US-$ 88.50
ISBN: 90-420-0516-5   Paper Hfl. 45,-/US-$ 25.50

Daniel Turner's prolific writings provide valuable insight into the practice
of a commonplace Enlightenment London surgeon. Examining his personal,
professional, and genteel achievements enhances our understanding of the
boundary between surgeons and physicians in Enlightenment 'marketplace'
practice. Turner's pioneering writing on skin disease, *De Morbis Cutaneis*,
emphasizes the skin's role as a physical and professional boundary between
university-educated physicians who treated internal disease and apprentice-
trained surgeons relegated to the care of external disorders. Turner also
argued that a pregnant woman's imagination could be transferred to her
unborn child, imprinting its skin with various marks and deformities. This
stance sparked a major pamphlet war between Turner and London physician
James Blondel, raising this phenomenon from a folk belief to a chief
concern of Enlightenment natural philosophy. Turner's career-long crusade
against quackery and his voluminous writings on syphilis, a common
'surgical' disorder, provide a refined view into distinctions between
orthodox and quack practices in 18th-Century London. Turner, long viewed
as a pioneer in British dermatology, also holds the Anglo-American
distinction of receiving a medical degree from Yale, the first such degree
offered from Colonial America.

------------------------------   *Editions Rodopi B.V.*

USA/Canada: 2015 South Park Place, Atlanta, GA 30339, Tel. (770)
933-0027, *Call toll-free* (U.S.only) 1-800-225-3998, Fax (770) 933-9644

All Other Countries: Tijnmuiden 7, 1046 AK Amsterdam, The Netherlands.
Tel. + + 31 (0)20 6114821, Fax + + 31 (0)20 4472979
          orders-queries@rodopi.nl — http://www.rodopi.nl

MEDICINE AND MODERN WARFARE

Ed. by Roger Cooter, Mark Harrison & Steve Sturdy

Amsterdam/Atlanta, GA 1999. X,286 pp.
(Clio Medica 55/The Wellcome Institute Series in the History of Medicine)

ISBN: 90-420-0546-7   Bound Hfl. 150,-/US-$ 83.-
ISBN: 90-420-0536-X   Paper Hfl. 45,-/US-$ 25.50

After years at the margins of medical history, the relationship between war and medicine is at last beginning to move centre-stage. The essays in this volume focus on one important aspect of that relationship: the practice and development of medicine within the armed forces from the late nineteenth century through to the end of the Second World War. During this crucial period, medicine came to occupy an important position in military life, especially during the two world wars when manpower was at a premium. Good medical provisions were vital to the conservation of manpower, protecting servicemen from disease and returning the sick and wounded to duty in the shortest possible time. A detailed knowledge of the serviceman's mind and body enabled the authorities to calculate and standardise rations, training and disciplinary procedures.

Spanning the laboratory and the battlefield, and covering a range of national contexts, the essays in this volume provide valuable insights into different national styles and priorities. They also examine the relationship between medical personnel and the armed forces as a whole, by looking at such matters as the prevention of disease, the treatment of psychiatric casualties and the development of medical science. The volume as a whole demonstrates that medicine became an increasingly important part of military life in the era of modern warfare, and suggests new avenues and approaches for future study.

---------------------------------   *Editions Rodopi B.V.*

USA/Canada: 2015 South Park Place, Atlanta, GA 30339, Tel. (770) 933-0027, *Call toll-free* (U.S.only) 1-800-225-3998, Fax (770) 933-9644

All Other Countries: Tijnmuiden 7, 1046 AK Amsterdam, The Netherlands. Tel. ++ 31 (0)20 6114821, Fax ++ 31 (0)20 4472979
         orders-queries@rodopi.nl —— http://www.rodopi.nl

PATHOLOGIES OF TRAVEL

Ed. by Richard Wrigley and George Revill

Amsterdam/Atlanta, GA 2000. XI,338 pp.
(Clio Medica 56/The Wellcome Institute Series in the History of Medicine)
ISBN: 90-420-0608-0   Bound Hfl. 160,-/US-$ 88.50
ISBN: 90-420-0598-X   Paper Hfl. 50,-/US-$ 27.50

The essays in this volume, which range across Europe, America and Africa, and from the 18th to the 20th centuries, argue that the experience of travel, and the business of representing that experience, involved an obligatory engagement with the disturbing perception that travel's pleasures were inseparable from its dangers and ennuis. Despite the confidence of some medical authorities in their recommendations of the therapeutic benefits to be derived from 'change of air' as a way of restoring a state of health, such opinions failed to establish a consensus, either amongst those who followed such peripatetic prescriptions, or amongst the medical professions in general. Mad doctors and climatologists alike were forced to adopt an essentially partisan stance in arguing their case for such recommendations, and were confronted by rival practitioners who could marshal counter-case histories which demonstrated diametrically opposed conclusions concerning the advisability of travel. To this extent, the history of travel and its pathologies is a particularly revealing instance of the way medical thinking was dependent on localised studies which might do more to challenge the universal applicability of generally accepted theories than they did to confirm their diagnostic reliability. The essays collected here not only contribute to our understanding of the conception and application of a variety of medical ideas, showing how they depended on beliefs about climate and corporeal constitution as well as often inconsistent data or récits culled from travellers and geographically dispersed case histories, but also open up illuminatingly complex perspectives on the uncertainties and dangers of the phenomenon of modern travel.

-------------------------------   *Editions Rodopi B.V.*

USA/Canada: 2015 South Park Place, Atlanta, GA 30339, Tel. (770) 933-0027, *Call toll-free* (U.S.only) 1-800-225-3998, Fax (770) 933-9644

All Other Countries: Tijnmuiden 7, 1046 AK Amsterdam, The Netherlands. Tel. ++ 31 (0)20 6114821, Fax ++ 31 (0)20 4472979
                orders-queries@rodopi.nl —— http://www.rodopi.nl

YUVAL LURIE

Cultural Beings.
Reading the Philosophers of *Genesis*

Amsterdam/Atlanta, GA 2000. VII,217 pp.
(Value Inquiry Book Series 89)
ISBN: 90-420-0469-X   Hfl. 70,-/US-$ 38.50

Human beings are a cultural species. This predicament enables them to take
on many different cultural identities, all of which transcend the bounds of
natural behavior of other species. To contemplate this predicament through
philosophy is to reflect on such questions as, What makes cultural forms of
life possible? What is encompassed in them? What lies at their core? What
distinguishes them from natural forms of life? What brings them about,
sustains, and causes them to change? Philosophical answers to these
questions predate abstract ways of thinking, as they are sometimes
embedded in ancient mythical and religious narratives. Such is the story
told in the first three chapters of the book of *Genesis* in the Bible, revealing
how human beings became the cultural beings that they are. This study
suggests how that ancient and most celebrated story in the literature of the
West may be read as harboring insightful philosophical observations on the
cultural nature of human beings. It first focuses on the very concept of
cultural forms of life, revealing its complicated conceptual links to natural
forms of life. It then offers an interpretive framework for reading mythical,
symbolic narratives. Using these ideas, it provides a philosophical reading
of the Biblical narrative, disclosing it to harbor a metaphysically oriented
conception of nature and two insightful philosophical overviews of the
cultural nature of human beings. Both overviews endow human beings with
an ability to manipulate nature, but in different ways: the first by
subjugating parcels of nature to human will; the second by subjugating
human beings themselves to a value-laden conception of things and ethical
forms of life. Thus, human beings are portrayed as natural creatures
possessed of a cultural nature that enables them to transform nature and
recreate themselves through their unique cultural predicament.

------------------------------   *Editions Rodopi B.V.*
USA/Canada: 2015 South Park Place, Atlanta, GA 30339, Tel. (770)
933-0027, *Call toll-free* (U.S.only) 1-800-225-3998, Fax (770) 933-9644

All Other Countries: Tijnmuiden 7, 1046 AK Amsterdam, The Netherlands.
Tel. + + 31 (0)20 6114821, Fax + + 31 (0)20 4472979
             orders-queries@rodopi.nl —— http://www.rodopi.nl

GARY J. ACQUAVIVA

Values, Violence, and Our Future

Amsterdam/Atlanta, GA 2000. IX, 208 pp.
(Value Inquiry Book Series 91)
ISBN: 90-420-0559-9   Hfl. 65,-/US-$ 36.-

This book identifies the character of human predators who violate others or themselves. The contagion of violence infects values that affect behavior. But we may call upon the intrinsic values of love, compassion, and creativity to oppose such violence. The book boldly argues for a renewal of the spiritual energy that gave rise to civilization.

-------------------------------------   *Editions Rodopi B.V.*

USA/Canada: 2015 South Park Place, Atlanta, GA 30339, Tel. (770) 933-0027, *Call toll-free* (U.S.only) 1-800-225-3998, Fax (770) 933-9644

All Other Countries: Tijnmuiden 7, 1046 AK Amsterdam, The Netherlands. Tel. ++ 31 (0)20 6114821, Fax ++ 31 (0)20 4472979
                orders-queries@rodopi.nl — http://www.rodopi.nl

ONE HUNDRED YEARS OF MASOCHISM
Literary Texts, Social and Cultural Contexts

Ed. by Michael C. Finke and Carl Niekerk

Amsterdam/Atlanta, GA 2000. VIII, 215 pp.
(Psychoanalysis and Culture 10)
ISBN: 90-420-0657-9   Hfl. 70,-/US-$ 38.50

Just over a century has passed since the sexologist Richard von Krafft-Ebing coined the term "masochism" in a revised edition of his *Psychopathia Sexualis* (1890). Put into circulation as part of the *fin-de-siècle* process through which sexuality and sexual practices considered deviant became medicalized, this suspicious concept grew in significance and explanatory power in the expanding new context of psychoanalytic discourse. Today the study of masochism shows signs of becoming a discipline in its own right, the political, social, and cultural ramifications of which exceed and, indeed, render problematic, traditional psychoanalytic perspectives on the phenomenon. The essays in this volume demonstrate, however, that the concept of masochism still offers a point of entry into psychoanalytic theory that, while revealing a number of its most vexing insufficiencies and problematic constructions, evokes also a sometimes surprising illuminative potential and capacity to adapt to changing social realities. And as the volume's title is meant to suggest, the authors represented here tend to agree that the continued rich viability of psychoanalytic theory in cultural analysis is best appreciated and ensured through engaging the theory's own social-historical and cultural contexts.
The volume includes clinical perspectives on masochism, and articles on medieval romance, Goethe, Sacher-Masoch, Krafft-Ebing's *Psychopathia Sexualis*, Turgenev, Tolstoy, Multatuli, Fassbinder, and masochism and postmodernism.

------------------------------   *Editions Rodopi B.V.*

USA/Canada: 6075 Roswell Rd., Ste. 219, Atlanta, GA 30328, Tel. (404) 843-4314, *Call toll-free* (U.S.only) 1-800-225-3998, Fax (404) 843-4315

All Other Countries: Tijnmuiden 7, 1046 AK Amsterdam, The Netherlands. Tel. ++ 31 (0)20 6114821, Fax ++ 31 (0)20 4472979
                orders-queries@rodopi.nl — http://www.rodopi.nl

JACQUES KRIEL

Matter, Mind, and Medicine
Transforming the Clinical Method

Amsterdam/Atlanta, GA 2000. XXXII,157 pp.
(Value Inquiry Book Series 93)
ISBN: 90-420-0799-0   Hfl. 70,-/US-$ 38.50

This book critically assesses the claim of modern medicine to scientific status, and it explores the implications of that claim for medicine's clinical method. Medicine models its scientific self-understanding on an obsolete positivist conception of science, reality, and consciousness. The body is viewed as a biological machine, disease as a breakdown of the machine, and therapy as the physical measures to fix that machine. Medicine's clinical method thus cannot deal with the full complexity of the ill human person. The book proposes a broader model of science and an alternative understanding of reality and of human consciousness which can become the basis of a transformed clinical method.

----------------------------------- *Editions Rodopi B.V.*

USA/Canada: 2015 South Park Place, Atlanta, GA 30339, Tel. (770) 933-0027, *Call toll-free* (U.S.only) 1-800-225-3998, Fax (770) 933-9644

All Other Countries: Tijnmuiden 7, 1046 AK Amsterdam, The Netherlands. Tel. + + 31 (0)20 6114821, Fax + + 31 (0)20 4472979
          orders-queries@rodopi.nl —— http://www.rodopi.nl

KATJA VERA TAVER

Johann Gottlieb Fichtes Wissenschaftslehre von 1810 Versuch einer Exegese

Amsterdam/Atlanta, GA 1999. XVIII,398 pp.
(Fichte-Studien Supplementa 12)
ISBN: 90-420-0679-X   Hfl. 140,-/US-$ 77.50

Johann Gottlieb Fichtes Spätwerk - versteht man hierunter die Wissenschaftslehren zwischen 1810 und 1814 - ist weitestgehend noch unbekannt. Die von Immanuel Hermann Fichte veröffentlichte Wissenschaftslehre von 1812, auf welche die Forschung sich gern abstützt, ist vom Herausgeber teils verfälscht, die Wissenschaftslehren von 1813 und 1814 blieben unvollendet. Erst jetzt ist die Wissenschftslehre von 1810, welche Einblick gibt in Fichtes spätes Denken, zugänglich geworden.

Dieses in der J.G. Fichte Gesamtausgabe inzwischen edierte Manuskript ist jedoch nur in einer mühsamen Exegese zu entschlüsseln, da es sich um ein nacktes Gerüst für die zu haltende Vorlesung handelt. So mußte der Originaltext von 1810 im Versuch einer getreuen Exegese gegliedert und unter Beiziehung späterer Schriften und insbesondere des vorangehenden Werkes Fichtes entschlüsselt, rekonstruiert und kommentiert werden. Dies erforderte den vorsichtigen Vorgriff auf die von Immanuel Hermann Fichte edierten späten Schriften sowie den Rückgriff auf die inzwischen in kritischer Edition vorliegenden frühen Schriften Fichtes, so die "Grundlage der gesamten Wissenschaftslehre" von 1794, sowie auf die das absolute Wissen thematisierende Wissenschaftslehre von 1801/02 aus Fichtes Umbruchzeit und die Beiziehung der Wissenschaftslehre von 1804 mit der "Anweisung zum seligen Leben" von 1806, welche Fichtes Spätphase einleiten und den Boden bilden, welchem Fichtes Spätwerk entsproß. Mitberücksichtigt wurde zur Wissenschaftslehre 1810 gehörende "Wissenschaftslehre in ihrem allgemeinen Umrisse", welche Fichte selbst als Rekapitulation für seine Hörer 1810 in Druck gegeben hatte, sowie die ebenfalls zum Druck bestimmten und 1817 erschienen "Thatsachen des Bewusstseyns" von 1810/11.

----------------------------   *Editions Rodopi B.V.*

USA/Canada: 2015 South Park Place, Atlanta, GA 30339, Tel. (770) 933-0027, *Call toll-free* (U.S.only) 1-800-225-3998, Fax (770) 933-9644

All Other Countries: Tijnmuiden 7, 1046 AK Amsterdam, The Netherlands. Tel. ++ 31 (0)20 6114821, Fax ++ 31 (0)20 4472979

BERNWARD LOHEIDE

Fichte und Novalis
Transzendentalphilosophisches Denken
im romantisierenden Diskurs

Amsterdam/Atlanta, GA 2000. 417 pp.
(Fichte-Studien Supplementa 13)
ISBN: 90-420-0689-7   Hfl. 130,-/US-$ 72.-

Die deutsche Romantik gilt gemeinhin als Überwindung der abstrakten Ich-Philosophie Fichtes. Gegen dieses weitverbreitete Klischee beweist die vorliegende Studie, daß das philosophische, naturwissenschaftliche und poetische Werk des Novalis auf genau diejenigen Probleme des Subjektdenkens antwortet, die Fichte zu einer Vertiefung seines eigenen Ansatzes bewegt haben. Kongenial greift Novalis diesen transzendentalen Ansatz seines Lehrers auf und nimmt damit zugleich in einigen Punkten dessen späte Wissenschaftslehre vorweg. Der Romantiker par excellende ist ein Fichteaner.

Editions Rodopi B.V.

USA/Canada: 2015 South Park Place, Atlanta, GA 30339, Tel. (770) 933-0027, *Call toll-free* (U.S.only) 1-800-225-3998, Fax (770) 933-9644

All Other Countries: Tijnmuiden 7, 1046 AK Amsterdam, The Netherlands. Tel. ++ 31 (0)20 6114821, Fax ++ 31 (0)20 4472979
orders-queries@rodopi.nl — http://www.rodopi.nl

THE MYSTERY OF VALUES
Studies in Axiology. Ludwig Grünberg

Ed. by Cornelia Grünberg and Laura Grünberg

Amsterdam/Atlanta, GA 2000. XVIII,157 pp.
(Value Inquiry Book Series 95)
ISBN: 90-420-0670-6   Hfl. 70,-/US-$ 38.50

This study of axiology explores the axiocentricity of being human. Human beings dwell in the realm of value. Values are not simply what persons have; values in large part are what persons are. The mystique of values is analyzed here in terms of their cultural, phenomenological, and ontological status. The relationship between science and values is debated. Values should not be submitted to reductionism. Postmodernism raises new problems for the future of a philosophy of values. Yet, we may direct our hopes toward happiness, universalism, and humanism as inseparable from value-life.

-------------------------------- *Editions Rodopi B.V.*

USA/Canada: 6075 Roswell Rd., Ste. 219, Atlanta, GA 30328, Tel. (404) 843-4314, *Call toll-free* (U.S.only) 1-800-225-3998, Fax (404) 843-4315

All Other Countries: Tijnmuiden 7, 1046 AK Amsterdam, The Netherlands. Tel. ++ 31 (0)20 6114821, Fax ++ 31 (0)20 4472979
      orders-queries@rodopi.nl —— http://www.rodopi.nl

LITERATURE AND HOMOSEXUALITY

Ed. by Michael J. Meyer

Amsterdam/Atlanta, GA 2000. VII,274 pp.
(Rodopi Perspectives on Modern Literature 21)
ISBN: 90-420-0529-7   Bound Hfl. 140,-/US-$ 80.50
ISBN: 90-420-0519-X   Paper Hfl. 45,-/US-$ 25.50

------------------------------   *Editions Rodopi B.V.*

USA/Canada: 6075 Roswell Rd., Ste. 219, Atlanta, GA 30328, Tel. (404) 843-4314, *Call toll-free* (U.S.only) 1-800-225-3998, Fax (404) 843-4315

All Other Countries: Tijnmuiden 7, 1046 AK Amsterdam, The Netherlands. Tel. ++ 31 (0)20 6114821, Fax ++ 31 (0)20 4472979
          orders-queries@rodopi.nl —— http://www.rodopi.nl

THE MORAL STATUS OF PERSONS
Perspectives on Bioethics

Ed. by Gerhold K. Becker

Amsterdam/Atlanta, GA 2000. VII,246 pp.
(Value Inquiry Book Series 96)
ISBN: 90-420-1201-3   Hfl. 100,-/US-$ 55.50

The advances in molecular biology and genetics, medicine and neurosciences, in ethology and environmental studies have put the concept of the person firmly on the philosophical agenda. Whereas earlier times seemed to have a clear understanding about the moral implications of personhood and its boundaries, today there is little consensus on such matters. Whether a patient in the last stages of Alzheimer's disease is still a person, or whether a human embryo is already a person are highly contentious issues.

This book tackles the issue of personhood and its moral implications head-on. The thirteen essays are representative of the major strands in the current bioethical debate and offer new insights into humanity's moral standing, its foundations, and its implications for social interaction. While most of the essays approach the issue by drawing on the rich intellectual tradition of the West, others offer a cross-cultural perspective and make available for ethical consideration the philosophical resources and the wisdom of the East. The contributors to this book are highly recognized philosophers, ethicists, theologians, and professionals in health care and medicine from East Asia (China, Japan), Europe, and North America.

The first part of the book probes the foundations of personhood. Examining critically the main theories on personhood in contemporary philosophy, the authors offer alternatives that better respond to contemporary challenges and their implications for bioethics.

The focus of the second part is firmly on the Confucian relational concept of the person and on the social constitution of personhood in traditional Japanese culture. While the essays challenge the individualistic features of personhood in the Western tradition, they lay the foundations for a richer concept that holds great promise for the resolution of moral dilemmas in modern medicine and health care.

The third part of the book enters into a dialogue with the Christian tradition and draws on its spiritual heritage in the search for answers to the contemporary challenges to human dignity and value. Its focus is on the Catholic social thought and Lutheran theology.

The fourth part addresses the moral status of persons in view of specific issues such as the effects of brain injury, gene therapy, and human cloning on personhood. It extends the scope of research beyond human beings and inquires also into the moral status of animals.

------------------------------   *Editions Rodopi B.V.*

USA/Canada: 6075 Roswell Rd., Ste. 219, Atlanta, GA 30328, Tel. (404) 843-4314, *Call toll-free* (U.S.only) 1-800-225-3998, Fax (404) 843-4315

All Other Countries: Tijnmuiden 7, 1046 AK Amsterdam, The Netherlands. Tel. ++ 31 (0)20 6114821, Fax ++ 31 (0)20 4472979
                    orders-queries@rodopi.nl —— http://www.rodopi.nl

www.ingramcontent.com/pod-product-compliance
Lightning Source LLC
Chambersburg PA
CBHW030646270326
41929CB00007B/233